Personal Healthcare Record

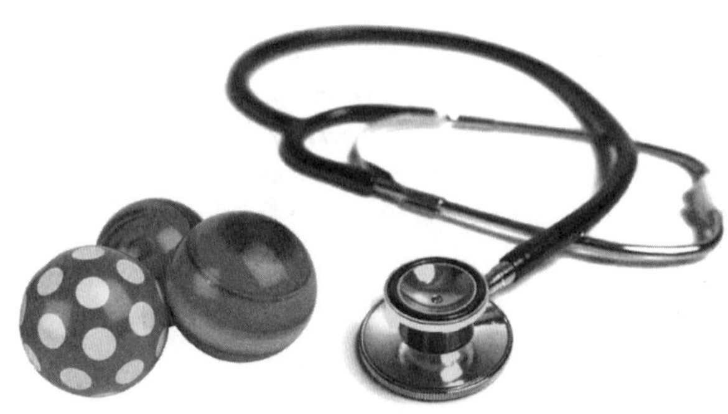

BIRTH TO SEVENTEEN YEARS OLD

For __________________________________
Name

From ____________ *to* ____________
Date *Date*

CONFIDENTIAL

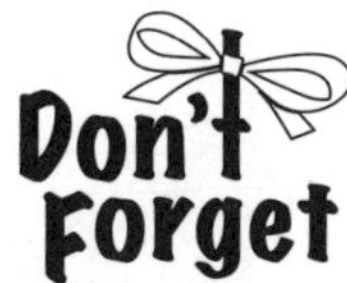

To buy additional copies or send comments, visit our website:

Website: www.PersonalHealthcareRecord.com

First Printing, 2011

Library of Congress Control Number: 2009940504

ISBN: 978-0-9744643-3-6

Tortuga Publishing
A Division of Tortuga Enterprises LLC
1142 S. Diamond Bar #261
CA 91765
United States of America

What they're saying....

"This is a vital gift for every new baby from every grandparent!" And adult children can do the same for their older adults whose healthcare gets more complicated every year. I especially appreciated the history charts—I am always filling them out, but forgetting the years and other details."
Kathleen L., Grandmother, Bellingham, WA

"…this would be a great tool for a parent to start for a child…As I fill out medical forms, I realize I can't recall exact dates and details of previous health conditions or treatments. Having everything in one location…trying to remember everything…this could have made everything so much easier. "
Shelley F., Baby Boomer, Phoenix, AZ

"The PHR finally motivated me to get my medical life in order. The thought of organizing my health records was daunting until I saw how the PHR did most of the work for me—add a few notes, staple some doctor's info. together and I was done! And it has been fun to track, which is easy now that all the info. is in one place."
Bill H., Carlsbad, CA

"We've all heard encouraging messages like 'take charge of your own healthcare or be a part of your healthcare team,' sending the message loud and clear that the most important person on your healthcare team is YOU! This PHR is the right tool for doing that! It's a means for organizing your healthcare information to keep you in charge—helping you connect the dots. There was a time when we could rely on doctors to do that; those days are gone."
Joseph S., Healthcare Consultant, South Jordan, UT

"The PHR is a valuable tool for everyone, ESPECIALLY in an emergency. Under extreme circumstances, time and proper diagnosis can make the difference between life and death. The ability to quickly access vital information from the patient, family member or caretaker can expedite the diagnosis process, saving valuable time. In a non-emergency situation, information is often lost in translation. A doctor's ability to treat is dependent on the history of the patient. Having the ability to view previous tests often eliminates the need to duplicate some tests. It also gives the physician a baseline for referencing changes in the patient's condition. I love my PHR and my family endorses it as well. Thanks!"
Susan C., CRT, Alta Loma, CA

"Most people struggle to remember symptoms and how they evolved over the course of treatment. Providing a tool that helps people be more disciplined about this process is a valuable service. Thank you!"
Susan H., Consultant, Oakland, CA

The Author's Story

The genesis for this journal came from a personal need. Over the past several years, I have faced a number of medical issues personally and within my family. To mention just a few, my mother was diagnosed with cancer and eventually passed away from Alzheimer's disease; my father had heart value replacement and a gangrenous gall bladder removed; my daughter incurred a serious neck injury, my sister was diagnosed and succumbed to cancer. My husband passed away unexpectedly from complications of a common surgery. His PHR was valuable in analyzing medical issues related to his death. I've had several medical situations that have led to surgeries and other treatments. It soon became very evident that a user-friendly system for organizing all these converging events was greatly needed. So, I began organizing all of our medical information to make it easier to keep everything and everyone's situations straight.

Along the way, I came to the conclusion that it made sense to begin this record at birth rather than in later life. While it's never too late to begin gathering and maintaining healthcare information, doing so earlier makes the information easier to collect and keep complete.

My initial efforts eventually inspired me to develop the this tool. I know that if you use this journal as intended, you will find it valuable too.

Take charge of your healthcare and best wishes for a long and healthy life!

Charla Hornung Spence

Dedication

To my husband, my mother and sister, Sally, now living with the angels.

Acknowledgements

Just as it takes a village to raise a child, it takes a team to publish a book. The PHR was truly a team effort and I must thank many for helping me develop this tool into something that will help people begin taking charge of their healthcare. I thank the healthcare professionals who evaluated and provided valuable input, particularly: Holly Ferguson, Physician Assistant; Susan Cuzynski, CRT. End-user consultants: Susan Harris, Bill Hornung, Joseph Stith, Shelley and John Fletcher, Kathleen Whiteside Langdon. I also thank Michael Adams who provided developmental critiques and editing services.; Antoinette and Jared Kurtiz, Strategies Literary Public Relations for their guidance and support in the publishing and marketing process; Lloyd Jassin for legal counsel; Gwyn Kennedy Snider for graphics; Meredith Gould for copy editing; and Brian Jud, Greg Snider and Amy Collins MacGregor for supporting distribution.

I wish to thank the Southern California Writers Association for their great industry speakers and much more. In my role as Secretary and Vice President of Membership, I have forged many friendships for which I am grateful.

I thank my family for their inspiration and support—my parents Charlotte and Bill, brother Bill, sister Lanna, husband Michael, daughter Jessica, and other family members and friends.

Contents

The contents of your Personal Healthcare Record are not designed to replace your doctors' healthcare advice or records. The PHR is intended to serve as an organizational aide only.

Foreword

Given the realities of today's healthcare and health insurance world, your child will likely have several different doctors, each of whom specialize in the treatment of any condition your child might develop. A Personal Healthcare Record (PHR) will help you navigate the healthcare terrain by providing important background and baseline information for the healthcare professionals you will visit. Maintained carefully and well, a PHR will help you prevent taking a lot of unnecessary or redundant steps that may cost money or, at the very least, time.

Charla Spence is the perfect person to develop the PHR because she is not a healthcare professional. She's a patient just like you who recognized the need for this valuable tool. She developed the PHR from the patient's point-of-view, using common terms to provide a practicable, portable organizational system for your healthcare history. Because this is not a medical reference book, only very basic medical information is included.

Introduction

Everyone should have a Personal Healthcare Record (PHR). Ideally, such an organizational system should begin at birth and be updated throughout your child's entire life. Many healthcare professionals and agencies encourage individuals to take charge of their health by following standard guidelines for diet, exercise, disease prevention and health maintenance. Now you have a handy, easy-to-use tool for tracking all this vital information!

Icons used in this book:

 Hints: helps you get the most value out of your PHR

 Caution: "must dos" to keep your PHR information up to date

 Note: important information that will be helpful to others

Benefits of keeping a PHR...

- READY-TO- GO The PHR reduces the thinking and time required for organizing this important information. Fill in the blanks, punch a few holes, and you're ready to go!

- PORTABLE This portable journal is easy to keep and transport. No need to access a computer or find the right software. No extra steps for entering constantly changing healthcare information. Add reports and comments on the spot! Sometimes the best technology is low technology!

- PERSONAL & FAMILY HISTORY When it's time for them to take responsibility for their own healthcare and records, hand your children their PHR and they'll have all of their healthcare history to date.

- CAREGIVER REFERENCE Relying on others to help care for your child? Trusted babysitters, caregivers, and family members can have healthcare records, along with a permission to treat, in case the need arises.

- IN CASE OF EMERGENCY In an emergency, any trusted person can grab your child's PHR and use it to answer all the inevitable questions. In the case of a natural disaster, computers may not work. Grab your PHR & have everything you will need!

 Note: *Make sure several trusted friends or family members know where you keep your PHR.*

How to Use This Journal

The PHR can be used in the bound book form; however, the PHR was developed for use in a 3-ring notebook format so that you can easily include additional pages, copies of medical tests, reports, etc. It also makes it easy to rearrange or move older documents to additional notebooks over time. The Healthcare History section and recent Journal pages should remain in the primary binder for easy reference by your healthcare providers, but since this is your child's journal feel free to rearrange it in whatever order makes sense to you. The icons are intended to draw your attention to important hints, notes or cautions.

Setting Up Your Child's PHR

✔ Remove the perforated pages, hole punch and place the contents in a 3-ring notebook. You may want to purchase a view type binder so you can put the covers and spine in the slip covers provided on the outside of the notebook.

✔ Insert tab dividers and pocket folders based on preference. These can be purchased at any office supply store.

✔ Carry a hole punch to make it easy to add, on the spot, any documents received from healthcare providers. Convenient notebook size three hole punches can be purchased from any office supply store.

 Hint: *Remember to keep all information in chronological (by the date) order to make it easy to reference. After setting up, move the Table of Contents and Introduction to the reference section.*

5 Simple Steps

To get the most from your PHR, please read and follow these 5 Simple Steps to get started.

1. Complete Healthcare History

Use Section B to capture information from the various healthcare sources as it becomes relevant and available. Work with your child's healthcare professionals to consolidate all healthcare history and other important information in one convenient place.

 Caution! *You must update the PHR with any new information when you get it.*

 Note: *Put Healthcare History at a Glance page and Permission to Treat in a page protector and make it the first page so that emergency personnel may find it quickly. Remove the wallet card page, cut to size indicated, complete information and place in your wallet for quick reference. Keep the wallet card in the template section so you can make new copies for future use.*

2. Prepare Journal Pages

Note or staple any new information from office visits and other updates onto your child's personal journal pages. Better yet, take the journal pages with you to make notes during each visit or other activity.

Even if your child does not have a healthcare appointment scheduled, you can begin to prepare for that event by collecting Concerns/Questions/Symptoms to discuss with your child's healthcare professional and then, note them on a journal page. Most healthcare professionals do appreciate serving patients who come prepared with a list of questions. Not only does this make the appointment time more efficient, but it will help you ensure that all your concerns and questions are addressed. There's also space on each Journal page to record vital signs. The following is a key for the vital signs on the Journal page:

Journal Key:

BP	– Blood Pressure	Gl	– Glucose
Ch	– Cholesterol	Rp	– Respirations
HR	– Heart Rate/Pulse	Tp	– Temperature
Ht	– Height	Wt	– Weight

Here are a few suggestions for making your visits to your healthcare professional more effective:

✓ Complete your child's PHR Journal page in advance of your child's appointment and take your PHR notebook with you. (See sample Journal Page on page 100)

 Hint: *If you're returning to one of your child's regular doctors, you may want to take only the current journal page, in a folder for privacy, rather than carry the entire PHR. This will also reduce the chances of losing your child's PHR or a stranger seeing confidential information.*

✓ When making your appointment, let the appointment desk receptionist know if you have several items to discuss with the doctor in addition to the primary reason for your appointment.

✓ Write down all information and actions from your child's visit on the Journal page.

 Hint: *You may prefer recording some of the information (like dental, hearing, vision or hospitalizations) on the optional pages 88-91 for quick reference and so that you do not have to dig for the information in the regular Journal pages.*

✓ Insert an extra page behind any forms where additional space is needed. Make extra copies of the general use page titled Symptom/Healthcare Event Journal located in the template section for this purpose.

 Caution: *Replace the Journal page and any related documents in the binder after your appointment so that the information is not misplaced.*

Note: *A convenient way for caregivers to help those who may attend appointments, with those being assisted, is to provide a list of questions on the journal page or insert an extra page with questions. Ask the healthcare professional to respond to the questions by writing answers directly on the journal page for your later reference.*

Remember, the ability for healthcare professionals to care for your child is only as good as your ability to provide accurate information!

3. Record Appointment Information

As soon as possible after your child's appointment, or preferably during the appointment, complete the Journal page with Diagnosis, Actions Needed and Outcome. This will enhance your ability to follow through on any actions you may need to take. If you need additional room to record the information from the visit, insert another page, or use another journal section to write your comments.

Hint: *Be sure to get a business card from healthcare professionals so you have all of their contact information. You may attach the business card or write the information on the Journal page in the box provided.*

4. Punch and Insert Materials

You will likely receive all types of reports and test results in different sizes. Rather than take the extra time to scan into an electronic system, simply punch holes in the document, place it behind the appropriate appointment in the Journal pages and you're done!

Hint: *For ease of use, move completed Journal pages to the back of the Journal Section so next appointment page is on top. This will keep the pages in date order without getting in your way.*

5. Schedule Future Healthcare

Based on your healthcare professionals recommendations, schedule the routine appointments like annual physicals, dental, hearing and vision check-ups.

Hint: *When needed, photocopy additional Journal pages and wallet cards from templates in Reference Section C. Do not write on the templates so that you can continue to make additional copies.*

SECTION A

Journal Pages

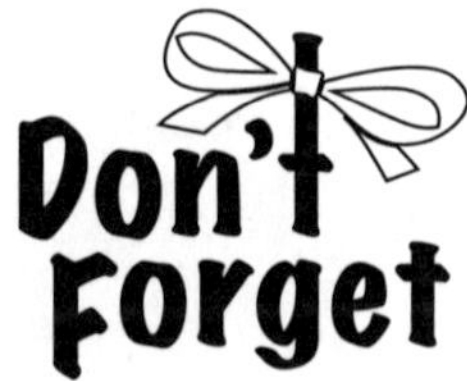

Personal Healthcare Record

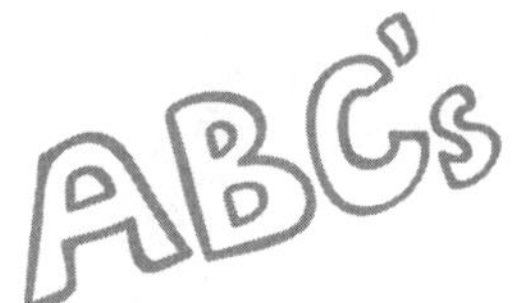

Personal Healthcare Record for: _______________________________________ *Page* _______

Healthcare Concern/Questions/Symptoms

Date _______________

____

____

____

____

____

____

____

____

Include relevant vital sign measurements as medical personnel complete your evaluation. (Reference key on page xi.)

BP _________   HR_________   Tp_________   Rp_________

HT_________   Wt_________   GL_________   Ch_________

Other _________________________________

____

Staple physician's or other healthcare provider's business card or write in contact information here.

Referred by:

____

Diagnosis

____

____

____

____

____

____

Actions Needed *(follow-up, referral, prescriptions, tests, etc.)*   Date Scheduled

____

____

____

____

Outcome

____

____

____

____

Healthcare Concern/Questions/Symptoms

Date ________________

____

____

____

____

____

____

____

Staple physician's or other healthcare provider's business card or write in contact information here.

Referred by:

____

Diagnosis

Include relevant vital sign measurements as medical personnel complete your evaluation. (Reference key on page xi.)

BP __________   HR__________   Tp__________   Rp__________

HT__________   Wt__________   GL__________   Ch__________

Other ____

____

____

____

____

____

____

Actions Needed *(follow-up, referral, prescriptions, tests, etc.)*

Date Scheduled

____

____

____

____

Outcome

____

____

____

____

Healthcare Concern/Questions/Symptoms

Date __________

____

____

____

____

____

____

____

Staple physician's or other healthcare provider's business card or write in contact information here.

Referred by:

____

Include relevant vital sign measurements as medical personnel complete your evaluation. (Reference key on page xi.)

BP__________   HR__________   Tp__________   Rp__________

HT__________   Wt__________   GL__________   Ch__________

Other ____

____

Diagnosis

____

____

____

____

____

____

Actions Needed *(follow-up, referral, prescriptions, tests, etc.)*   Date Scheduled

____

____

____

____

Outcome

____

____

____

____

Personal Healthcare Record for: ____ *Page* ___________

Healthcare Concern/Questions/Symptoms

Date ________________

____

____

____

____

____

____

____

____

Include relevant vital sign measurements as medical personnel complete your evaluation. (Reference key on page xi.)

BP __________   HR__________   Tp__________   Rp__________

HT__________   Wt__________   GL__________   Ch__________

Other ____

____

____

Diagnosis

____

____

____

____

____

____

____

Actions Needed *(follow-up, referral, prescriptions, tests, etc.)*   Date Scheduled

____

____

____

____

Outcome

____

____

____

____

Healthcare Concern/Questions/Symptoms

Date ________________

____

____

____

____

____

____

____

Staple physician's or other healthcare provider's business card or write in contact information here.

Referred by:

____

Include relevant vital sign measurements as medical personnel complete your evaluation. (Reference key on page xi.)

BP __________ HR__________ Tp__________ Rp__________

HT__________ Wt__________ GL__________ Ch__________

Other ____________________________________

Diagnosis

____

____

____

____

____

Actions Needed *(follow-up, referral, prescriptions, tests, etc.)*   Date Scheduled

____

____

____

____

Outcome

____

____

____

____

Healthcare Concern/Questions/Symptoms

Date _________________

____

____

____

____

____

____

____

Include relevant vital sign measurements as medical personnel complete your evaluation. (Reference key on page xi.)

BP __________   HR__________   Tp__________   Rp__________

HT__________   Wt__________   GL__________   Ch__________

Other ______________________________________

____

Staple physician's or other healthcare provider's business card or write in contact information here.

Referred by:

____

Diagnosis

____

____

____

____

____

____

Actions Needed *(follow-up, referral, prescriptions, tests, etc.)*

Date Scheduled

____

____

____

____

Outcome

____

____

____

____

Healthcare Concern/Questions/Symptoms

Date __________

____

____

____

____

____

____

Staple physician's or other healthcare provider's business card or write in contact information here.

Referred by:

____

Include relevant vital sign measurements as medical personnel complete your evaluation. (Reference key on page xi.)

BP __________ HR__________ Tp__________ Rp__________

HT__________ Wt__________ GL__________ Ch__________

Other ____

____

Diagnosis

____

____

____

____

____

____

Actions Needed *(follow-up, referral, prescriptions, tests, etc.)*   Date Scheduled

____

____

____

____

Outcome

____

____

____

____

Healthcare Concern/Questions/Symptoms

Date _______________

____

____

____

____

____

____

____

Include relevant vital sign measurements as medical personnel complete your evaluation. (Reference key on page xi.)

BP _________   HR_________   Tp_________   Rp_________

HT_________   Wt_________   GL_________   Ch_________

Other _________________________________

____

Staple physician's or other healthcare provider's business card or write in contact information here.

Referred by:

____

Diagnosis

____

____

____

____

____

____

Actions Needed *(follow-up, referral, prescriptions, tests, etc.)*

Date Scheduled

____

____

____

____

Outcome

____

____

____

____

Healthcare Concern/Questions/Symptoms

Date _________________

____

____

____

____

____

____

Staple physician's or other healthcare provider's business card or write in contact information here.

Referred by:

____

Include relevant vital sign measurements as medical personnel complete your evaluation. (Reference key on page xi.)

BP __________   HR__________   Tp__________   Rp__________

HT__________   Wt__________   GL__________   Ch__________

Other _______________________________

____

Diagnosis

____

____

____

____

____

Actions Needed *(follow-up, referral, prescriptions, tests, etc.)*   Date Scheduled

____

____

____

____

Outcome

____

____

____

____

Personal Healthcare Record for: ____   *Page* _________

Healthcare Concern/Questions/Symptoms

Date _________________

____

____

____

____

____

____

____

Include relevant vital sign measurements as medical personnel complete your evaluation. (Reference key on page xi.)

BP _________   HR_________   Tp_________   Rp_________

HT_________   Wt_________   GL_________   Ch_______

Other _______________________________________

____

Staple physician's or other healthcare provider's business card or write in contact information here.

Referred by:

____

Diagnosis

____

____

____

____

____

____

Actions Needed *(follow-up, referral, prescriptions, tests, etc.)*

Date Scheduled

____

____

____

____

Outcome

____

____

____

____

Healthcare Concern/Questions/Symptoms

Date __________________

____

Staple physician's or other healthcare provider's business card or write in contact information here.

Referred by:

____

Include relevant vital sign measurements as medical personnel complete your evaluation. (Reference key on page xi.)

BP __________   HR__________   Tp__________   Rp__________

HT__________   Wt__________   GL__________   Ch__________

Other ____

Diagnosis

Actions Needed *(follow-up, referral, prescriptions, tests, etc.)*

Date Scheduled

Outcome

Healthcare Concern/Questions/Symptoms

Date ___________________

____

____

____

____

____

____

____

Staple physician's or other healthcare provider's business card or write in contact information here.

Referred by:

____

Include relevant vital sign measurements as medical personnel complete your evaluation. (Reference key on page xi.)

BP __________   HR__________   Tp__________   Rp__________

HT__________   Wt__________   GL__________   Ch__________

Other __________________________________

____

Diagnosis

____

____

____

____

____

____

Actions Needed *(follow-up, referral, prescriptions, tests, etc.)*   Date Scheduled

____

____

____

____

Outcome

____

____

____

____

Healthcare Concern/Questions/Symptoms

Date _______________

____

____

____

____

____

____

____

Include relevant vital sign measurements as medical personnel complete your evaluation. (Reference key on page xi.)

BP __________ HR__________ Tp__________ Rp__________

HT__________ Wt__________ GL__________ Ch__________

Other ____

____

> Staple physician's or other healthcare provider's business card or write in contact information here.
>
> Referred by:
>
> ____

Diagnosis

____

____

____

____

____

____

Actions Needed *(follow-up, referral, prescriptions, tests, etc.)*   Date Scheduled

____

____

____

____

Outcome

____

____

____

____

Healthcare Concern/Questions/Symptoms

Date ________________

____

____

____

____

____

____

____

> Staple physician's or other healthcare provider's business card or write in contact information here.
>
> Referred by:
>
> ________________________________

Include relevant vital sign measurements as medical personnel complete your evaluation. (Reference key on page xi.)

BP __________   HR __________   Tp __________   Rp __________

HT __________   Wt __________   GL __________   Ch __________

Other ____

Diagnosis

____

____

____

____

____

____

____

Actions Needed *(follow-up, referral, prescriptions, tests, etc.)*   Date Scheduled

____

____

____

____

Outcome

____

____

____

____

Personal Healthcare Record for: ____ *Page* _________

Healthcare Concern/Questions/Symptoms

Date _______________

____

____

____

____

____

____

____

Include relevant vital sign measurements as medical personnel complete your evaluation. (Reference key on page xi.)

BP _________   HR_________   Tp_________   Rp_________

HT_________   Wt_________   GL_________   Ch_________

Other _______________________________________

____

Staple physician's or other healthcare provider's business card or write in contact information here.

Referred by:

____

Diagnosis

____

____

____

____

____

____

Actions Needed *(follow-up, referral, prescriptions, tests, etc.)*   Date Scheduled

____

____

____

____

Outcome

____

____

____

____

Healthcare Concern/Questions/Symptoms

Date _____________

____

____

____

____

____

____

____

____

Include relevant vital sign measurements as medical personnel complete your evaluation. (Reference key on page xi.)

BP __________   HR__________   Tp__________   Rp__________

HT__________   Wt__________   GL__________   Ch__________

Other ____________________________________

____

Staple physician's or other healthcare provider's business card or write in contact information here.

Referred by:

____

Diagnosis

____

____

____

____

____

____

Actions Needed *(follow-up, referral, prescriptions, tests, etc.)*   Date Scheduled

____

____

____

____

Outcome

____

____

____

____

Healthcare Concern/Questions/Symptoms

Date _______________

____

____

____

____

____

____

____

Staple physician's or other healthcare provider's business card or write in contact information here.

Referred by:

____

Include relevant vital sign measurements as medical personnel complete your evaluation. (Reference key on page xi.)

BP __________ HR__________ Tp__________ Rp__________

HT__________ Wt__________ GL __________ Ch __________

Other _______________________________________

____

Diagnosis

____

____

____

____

____

____

Actions Needed *(follow-up, referral, prescriptions, tests, etc.)*   Date Scheduled

____

____

____

____

Outcome

____

____

____

____

Healthcare Concern/Questions/Symptoms

Date __________________

____

____

____

____

____

____

____

Include relevant vital sign measurements as medical personnel complete your evaluation. (Reference key on page xi.)

BP __________ HR__________ Tp__________ Rp__________

HT__________ Wt__________ GL__________ Ch__________

Other ____

____

Staple physician's or other healthcare provider's business card or write in contact information here.

Referred by:

____

Diagnosis

____

____

____

____

____

____

Actions Needed *(follow-up, referral, prescriptions, tests, etc.)*   Date Scheduled

____

____

____

____

Outcome

____

____

____

____

Personal Healthcare Record for: ____ *Page* ___________

Healthcare Concern/Questions/Symptoms

Date ________________

____

____

____

____

____

____

____

Include relevant vital sign measurements as medical personnel complete your evaluation. (Reference key on page xi.)

BP __________ HR__________ Tp__________ Rp__________

HT__________ Wt__________ GL__________ Ch__________

Other _______________________________________

____

____

Diagnosis

____

____

____

____

____

____

____

Actions Needed *(follow-up, referral, prescriptions, tests, etc.)*   Date Scheduled

____

____

____

____

Outcome

____

____

____

____

Healthcare Concern/Questions/Symptoms

Date ___________________

____

____

____

____

____

____

____

Staple physician's or other healthcare provider's business card or write in contact information here.

Referred by:

____

Include relevant vital sign measurements as medical personnel complete your evaluation. (Reference key on page xi.)

BP __________   HR __________   Tp __________   Rp __________

HT __________   Wt __________   GL __________   Ch __________

Other ____

____

Diagnosis

____

____

____

____

____

____

Actions Needed *(follow-up, referral, prescriptions, tests, etc.)*   Date Scheduled

____

____

____

Outcome

____

____

____

____

Healthcare Concern/Questions/Symptoms

Date _______________

____

____

____

____

____

____

____

Include relevant vital sign measurements as medical personnel complete your evaluation. (Reference key on page xi.)

BP __________ HR__________ Tp__________ Rp__________

HT__________ Wt__________ GL__________ Ch__________

Other _______________________________

____

Staple physician's or other healthcare provider's business card or write in contact information here.

Referred by:

____

Diagnosis

____

____

____

____

____

____

Actions Needed *(follow-up, referral, prescriptions, tests, etc.)*　　　　Date Scheduled

____

____

____

____

Outcome

____

____

____

____

Healthcare Concern/Questions/Symptoms

Date _______________

____

____

____

____

____

____

____

Staple physician's or other healthcare provider's business card or write in contact information here.

Referred by:

____

Include relevant vital sign measurements as medical personnel complete your evaluation. (Reference key on page xi.)

BP __________   HR _________   Tp _________   Rp _________

HT _________   Wt _________   GL _________   Ch _________

Other _____________________________________

____

Diagnosis

____

____

____

____

____

Actions Needed *(follow-up, referral, prescriptions, tests, etc.)*   Date Scheduled

____

____

____

____

Outcome

____

____

____

____

Healthcare Concern/Questions/Symptoms

Date ________________

____

____

____

____

____

____

____

> Staple physician's or other healthcare provider's business card or write in contact information here.
>
> Referred by:
>
> ________________________________

Include relevant vital sign measurements as medical personnel complete your evaluation. (Reference key on page xi.)

BP ___________ HR___________ Tp___________ Rp___________

HT___________ Wt___________ GL___________ Ch___________

Other ________________________________

____

Diagnosis

____

____

____

____

____

____

Actions Needed *(follow-up, referral, prescriptions, tests, etc.)*   Date Scheduled

____

____

____

____

Outcome

____

____

____

____

Healthcare Concern/Questions/Symptoms

Date ________________

____

____

____

____

____

____

____

Staple physician's or other healthcare provider's business card or write in contact information here.

Referred by:

____

Include relevant vital sign measurements as medical personnel complete your evaluation. (Reference key on page xi.)

BP __________   HR__________   Tp__________   Rp__________

HT__________   Wt__________   GL__________   Ch__________

Other ____

____

Diagnosis

____

____

____

____

____

____

Actions Needed *(follow-up, referral, prescriptions, tests, etc.)*   Date Scheduled

____

____

____

____

Outcome

____

____

____

____

Healthcare Concern/Questions/Symptoms

Date ________________

____

____

____

____

____

____

____

Staple physician's or other healthcare provider's business card or write in contact information here.

Referred by:

____

Include relevant vital sign measurements as medical personnel complete your evaluation. (Reference key on page xi.)

BP __________   HR__________   Tp__________   Rp__________

HT__________   Wt__________   GL__________   Ch__________

Other ____

____

Diagnosis

____

____

____

____

____

____

Actions Needed *(follow-up, referral, prescriptions, tests, etc.)*   Date Scheduled

____

____

____

____

Outcome

____

____

____

____

Healthcare Concern/Questions/Symptoms

Date _______________

____
____
____
____
____
____

Staple physician's or other healthcare provider's business card or write in contact information here.

Referred by:

____

Include relevant vital sign measurements as medical personnel complete your evaluation. (Reference key on page xi.)

BP _________   HR _________   Tp _________   Rp _________

HT _________   Wt _________   GL _________   Ch _________

Other _______________________________________
____

Diagnosis

____
____
____
____
____
____

Actions Needed *(follow-up, referral, prescriptions, tests, etc.)*   Date Scheduled

____
____
____
____

Outcome

____
____
____
____

Healthcare Concern/Questions/Symptoms

Date _______________

____

____

____

____

____

____

____

Include relevant vital sign measurements as medical personnel complete your evaluation. (Reference key on page xi.)

BP __________   HR__________   Tp__________   Rp__________

HT__________   Wt__________   GL__________   Ch__________

Other __________________________________

____

Staple physician's or other healthcare provider's business card or write in contact information here.

Referred by:

____

Diagnosis

____

____

____

____

____

____

Actions Needed *(follow-up, referral, prescriptions, tests, etc.)*   Date Scheduled

____

____

____

____

Outcome

____

____

____

____

Healthcare Concern/Questions/Symptoms

Date _________________

____

____

____

____

____

____

____

Staple physician's or other healthcare provider's business card or write in contact information here.

Referred by:

____

Include relevant vital sign measurements as medical personnel complete your evaluation. (Reference key on page xi.)

BP _________   HR_________   Tp_________   Rp_________

HT_________   Wt_________   GL_________   Ch_________

Other _________________________________

____

Diagnosis

____

____

____

____

____

____

Actions Needed *(follow-up, referral, prescriptions, tests, etc.)*   Date Scheduled

____

____

____

____

Outcome

____

____

____

____

Healthcare Concern/Questions/Symptoms

Date _______________

____

____

____

____

____

____

____

Staple physician's or other healthcare provider's business card or write in contact information here.

Referred by:

____

Include relevant vital sign measurements as medical personnel complete your evaluation. (Reference key on page xi.)

BP _________ HR _________ Tp _________ Rp _________

HT _________ Wt _________ GL _________ Ch _________

Other _______________________________________

____

Diagnosis

____

____

____

____

____

____

Actions Needed *(follow-up, referral, prescriptions, tests, etc.)*   Date Scheduled

____

____

____

____

Outcome

____

____

____

____

Healthcare Concern/Questions/Symptoms

Date _______________

____

____

____

____

____

____

____

Staple physician's or other healthcare provider's business card or write in contact information here.

Referred by:

____

Diagnosis

Include relevant vital sign measurements as medical personnel complete your evaluation. (Reference key on page xi.)

BP __________ HR__________ Tp__________ Rp__________

HT__________ Wt__________ GL__________ Ch__________

Other __________________________________

____

____

____

____

____

____

____

Actions Needed *(follow-up, referral, prescriptions, tests, etc.)*   Date Scheduled

____

____

____

____

Outcome

____

____

____

____

Healthcare Concern/Questions/Symptoms

Date ________________

____

____

____

____

____

____

____

Staple physician's or other healthcare provider's business card or write in contact information here.

Referred by:

____

Include relevant vital sign measurements as medical personnel complete your evaluation. (Reference key on page xi.)

BP ___________   HR___________   Tp___________   Rp___________

HT___________   Wt___________   GL___________   Ch___________

Other _______________________________________

____

Diagnosis

____

____

____

____

____

____

____

Actions Needed *(follow-up, referral, prescriptions, tests, etc.)*   Date Scheduled

____

____

____

____

Outcome

____

____

____

____

Healthcare Concern/Questions/Symptoms

Date __________________

Staple physician's or other healthcare provider's business card or write in contact information here.

Referred by:

____

Include relevant vital sign measurements as medical personnel complete your evaluation. (Reference key on page xi.)

BP __________   HR __________   Tp __________   Rp __________

HT __________   Wt __________   GL __________   Ch __________

Other _______________________________________

Diagnosis

Actions Needed *(follow-up, referral, prescriptions, tests, etc.)*   Date Scheduled

Outcome

Healthcare Concern/Questions/Symptoms

Date ________________

____

____

____

____

____

____

____

Staple physician's or other healthcare provider's business card or write in contact information here.

Referred by:

____

Include relevant vital sign measurements as medical personnel complete your evaluation. (Reference key on page xi.)

BP __________   HR__________   Tp__________   Rp__________

HT__________   Wt__________   GL__________   Ch__________

Other ____

Diagnosis

____

____

____

____

____

____

Actions Needed *(follow-up, referral, prescriptions, tests, etc.)*   Date Scheduled

____

____

____

____

Outcome

____

____

____

____

Healthcare Concern/Questions/Symptoms

Date __________________

____

____

____

____

____

____

____

____

Staple physician's or other healthcare provider's business card or write in contact information here.

Referred by:

____

Include relevant vital sign measurements as medical personnel complete your evaluation. (Reference key on page xi.)

BP __________   HR__________   Tp__________   Rp__________

HT__________   Wt__________   GL__________   Ch__________

Other _______________________________________

____

Diagnosis

____

____

____

____

____

____

Actions Needed *(follow-up, referral, prescriptions, tests, etc.)*

Date Scheduled

____

____

____

____

Outcome

____

____

____

____

Healthcare Concern/Questions/Symptoms

Date ________________

____

____

____

____

____

____

____

____

> Staple physician's or other healthcare provider's business card or write in contact information here.
>
> Referred by:
>
> ________________________________

Include relevant vital sign measurements as medical personnel complete your evaluation. (Reference key on page xi.)

BP __________   HR__________   Tp__________   Rp__________

HT__________   Wt__________   GL__________   Ch__________

Other __________________________________

____

Diagnosis

____

____

____

____

____

____

Actions Needed *(follow-up, referral, prescriptions, tests, etc.)*   Date Scheduled

____

____

____

____

Outcome

____

____

____

____

Healthcare Concern/Questions/Symptoms

Date _____________

____

____

____

____

____

____

> Staple physician's or other healthcare provider's business card or write in contact information here.
>
> Referred by:
>
> ____

Include relevant vital sign measurements as medical personnel complete your evaluation. (Reference key on page xi.)

BP _________   HR _________   Tp _________   Rp _________

HT _________   Wt _________   GL _________   Ch _________

Other _____________________________________

____

Diagnosis

____

____

____

____

____

____

Actions Needed *(follow-up, referral, prescriptions, tests, etc.)*

Date Scheduled

____

____

____

____

Outcome

____

____

____

____

Healthcare Concern/Questions/Symptoms

Date _________________

____

____

____

____

____

____

____

Staple physician's or other healthcare provider's business card or write in contact information here.

Referred by:

____

Include relevant vital sign measurements as medical personnel complete your evaluation. (Reference key on page xi.)

BP _________   HR_________   Tp_________   Rp_________

HT_________   Wt_________   GL_________   Ch_________

Other _______________________________________

____

Diagnosis

____

____

____

____

____

____

Actions Needed *(follow-up, referral, prescriptions, tests, etc.)*   Date Scheduled

____

____

____

____

Outcome

____

____

____

____

Healthcare Concern/Questions/Symptoms

Date _________________

____

____

____

____

____

____

____

> Staple physician's or other healthcare provider's business card or write in contact information here.
>
> Referred by:
>
> _______________________________

Include relevant vital sign measurements as medical personnel complete your evaluation. (Reference key on page xi.)

BP _________ HR_________ Tp _________ Rp_________

HT _________ Wt_________ GL _________ Ch _________

Other _________________________________

____

Diagnosis

____

____

____

____

____

____

____

Actions Needed *(follow-up, referral, prescriptions, tests, etc.)*

Date Scheduled

____

____

____

____

Outcome

____

____

____

____

Healthcare Concern/Questions/Symptoms

Date ________________

____

____

____

____

____

____

____

Include relevant vital sign measurements as medical personnel complete your evaluation. (Reference key on page xi.)

BP _________ HR_________ Tp_________ Rp_________

HT_________ Wt_________ GL_________ Ch_________

Other _________________________________

____

Staple physician's or other healthcare provider's business card or write in contact information here.

Referred by:

____

Diagnosis

____

____

____

____

____

____

____

Actions Needed *(follow-up, referral, prescriptions, tests, etc.)*

Date Scheduled

____

____

____

____

Outcome

____

____

____

____

Healthcare Concern/Questions/Symptoms

Date _______________

____

____

____

____

____

____

____

Staple physician's or other healthcare provider's business card or write in contact information here.

Referred by:

____

Include relevant vital sign measurements as medical personnel complete your evaluation. (Reference key on page xi.)

BP _________   HR _________   Tp _________   Rp _________

HT _________   Wt _________   GL _________   Ch _________

Other _______________________________________

____

Diagnosis

____

____

____

____

____

____

____

Actions Needed *(follow-up, referral, prescriptions, tests, etc.)*   Date Scheduled

____

____

____

____

Outcome

____

____

____

____

____

Healthcare Concern/Questions/Symptoms

Date _______________

____

____

____

____

____

____

____

Staple physician's or other healthcare provider's business card or write in contact information here.

Referred by:

____

Include relevant vital sign measurements as medical personnel complete your evaluation. (Reference key on page xi.)

BP _________   HR_________   Tp_________   Rp_________

HT_________   Wt_________   GL _________   Ch_________

Other ____

____

Diagnosis

____

____

____

____

____

____

Actions Needed *(follow-up, referral, prescriptions, tests, etc.)*   Date Scheduled

____

____

____

____

Outcome

____

____

____

____

Healthcare Concern/Questions/Symptoms

Date ________________

____

____

____

____

____

____

____

Staple physician's or other healthcare provider's business card or write in contact information here.

Referred by:

____

Include relevant vital sign measurements as medical personnel complete your evaluation. (Reference key on page xi.)

BP _________   HR _________   Tp _________   Rp _________

HT _________   Wt _________   GL _________   Ch _________

Other _____________________________________

____

Diagnosis

____

____

____

____

____

____

Actions Needed *(follow-up, referral, prescriptions, tests, etc.)*   Date Scheduled

____

____

____

____

Outcome

____

____

____

____

Healthcare Concern/Questions/Symptoms

Date _______________

____

____

____

____

____

____

____

____

Staple physician's or other healthcare provider's business card or write in contact information here.

Referred by:

____

Diagnosis

____

____

____

____

____

____

Include relevant vital sign measurements as medical personnel complete your evaluation. (Reference key on page xi.)

BP _________   HR _________   Tp _________   Rp _________

HT _________   Wt _________   GL _________   Ch _________

Other _________________________________

Actions Needed *(follow-up, referral, prescriptions, tests, etc.)*   Date Scheduled

____

____

____

____

Outcome

____

____

____

____

Healthcare Concern/Questions/Symptoms

Date _________________

____

____

____

____

____

____

____

Include relevant vital sign measurements as medical personnel complete your evaluation. (Reference key on page xi.)

BP _________   HR _________   Tp _________   Rp _________

HT _________   Wt _________   GL _________   Ch _________

Other _________________________________

____

Staple physician's or other healthcare provider's business card or write in contact information here.

Referred by:

____

Diagnosis

____

____

____

____

____

____

Actions Needed *(follow-up, referral, prescriptions, tests, etc.)*   Date Scheduled

____

____

____

____

Outcome

____

____

____

____

Healthcare Concern/Questions/Symptoms

Date _______________

____

____

____

____

____

____

____

> *Staple physician's or other healthcare provider's business card or write in contact information here.*
>
> Referred by:
>
> _______________________________________

Include relevant vital sign measurements as medical personnel complete your evaluation. (Reference key on page xi.)

BP __________   HR__________   Tp__________   Rp__________

HT__________   Wt__________   GL__________   Ch__________

Other   ____

____

Diagnosis

____

____

____

____

____

____

Actions Needed *(follow-up, referral, prescriptions, tests, etc.)*   Date Scheduled

____

____

____

____

Outcome

____

____

____

____

Personal Healthcare Record for: ____ *Page* ___________

Healthcare Concern/Questions/Symptoms

Date ________________

____

____

____

____

____

____

____

____

Include relevant vital sign measurements as medical personnel complete your evaluation. (Reference key on page xi.)

BP __________   HR __________   Tp __________   Rp __________

HT __________   Wt __________   GL __________   Ch __________

Other ____

____

Staple physician's or other healthcare provider's business card or write in contact information here.

Referred by:

____

Diagnosis

____

____

____

____

____

____

Actions Needed *(follow-up, referral, prescriptions, tests, etc.)*   Date Scheduled

____

____

____

____

Outcome

____

____

____

____

Healthcare Concern/Questions/Symptoms

Date _______________

____

____

____

____

____

____

Staple physician's or other healthcare provider's business card or write in contact information here.

Referred by:

____

Include relevant vital sign measurements as medical personnel complete your evaluation. (Reference key on page xi.)

BP ___________   HR___________   Tp___________   Rp___________

HT___________   Wt___________   GL___________   Ch___________

Other _______________________________________

____

Diagnosis

____

____

____

____

____

____

Actions Needed *(follow-up, referral, prescriptions, tests, etc.)*   Date Scheduled

____

____

____

____

Outcome

____

____

____

____

Healthcare Concern/Questions/Symptoms

Date _______________

____

____

____

____

____

____

____

Staple physician's or other healthcare provider's business card or write in contact information here.

Referred by:

____

Include relevant vital sign measurements as medical personnel complete your evaluation. (Reference key on page xi.)

BP _________   HR _________   Tp _________   Rp _________

HT _________   Wt _________   GL _________   Ch _________

Other _____________________________________

____

Diagnosis

____

____

____

____

____

____

Actions Needed *(follow-up, referral, prescriptions, tests, etc.)*

Date Scheduled

____

____

____

____

Outcome

____

____

____

____

Healthcare Concern/Questions/Symptoms

Date __________________

____

____

____

____

____

____

Staple physician's or other healthcare provider's business card or write in contact information here.

Referred by:

____

Include relevant vital sign measurements as medical personnel complete your evaluation. (Reference key on page xi.)

BP __________   HR__________   Tp__________   Rp__________

HT__________   Wt__________   GL__________   Ch__________

Other ____

Diagnosis

____

____

____

____

____

____

Actions Needed *(follow-up, referral, prescriptions, tests, etc.)*

Date Scheduled

____

____

____

____

Outcome

____

____

____

____

Healthcare Concern/Questions/Symptoms

Date __________________

____

____

____

____

____

____

Staple physician's or other healthcare provider's business card or write in contact information here.

Referred by:

____

Include relevant vital sign measurements as medical personnel complete your evaluation. (Reference key on page xi.)

BP __________   HR__________   Tp__________   Rp__________

HT__________   Wt__________   GL__________   Ch__________

Other ______________________________________

____

Diagnosis

____

____

____

____

____

____

____

Actions Needed *(follow-up, referral, prescriptions, tests, etc.)*   Date Scheduled

____

____

____

____

Outcome

____

____

____

____

Healthcare Concern/Questions/Symptoms

Date _______________

____

____

____

____

____

____

____

Staple physician's or other healthcare provider's business card or write in contact information here.

Referred by:

____

Diagnosis

Include relevant vital sign measurements as medical personnel complete your evaluation. (Reference key on page xi.)

BP __________ HR__________ Tp__________ Rp__________

HT__________ Wt__________ GL__________ Ch__________

Other ___________________________________

____

____

____

____

____

____

____

____

Actions Needed *(follow-up, referral, prescriptions, tests, etc.)*   Date Scheduled

____

____

____

____

Outcome

____

____

____

____

Personal Healthcare Record for: ____ *Page* __________

Healthcare Concern/Questions/Symptoms

Date _______________

____

____

____

____

____

____

Staple physician's or other healthcare provider's business card or write in contact information here.

Referred by:

____

Include relevant vital sign measurements as medical personnel complete your evaluation. (Reference key on page xi.)

BP __________   HR__________   Tp__________   Rp__________

HT __________   Wt__________   GL __________   Ch __________

Other ____

____

Diagnosis

____

____

____

____

____

____

Actions Needed *(follow-up, referral, prescriptions, tests, etc.)*

Date Scheduled

____

____

____

____

Outcome

____

____

____

____

Healthcare Concern/Questions/Symptoms

Date _______________

____

____

____

____

____

____

____

Staple physician's or other healthcare provider's business card or write in contact information here.

Referred by:

____

Include relevant vital sign measurements as medical personnel complete your evaluation. (Reference key on page xi.)

BP __________   HR__________   Tp__________   Rp__________

HT__________   Wt__________   GL__________   Ch__________

Other _______________________________

Diagnosis

____

____

____

____

____

____

Actions Needed *(follow-up, referral, prescriptions, tests, etc.)*   Date Scheduled

____

____

____

____

Outcome

____

____

____

____

Healthcare Concern/Questions/Symptoms

Date ___________________

____

____

____

____

____

____

____

Staple physician's or other healthcare provider's business card or write in contact information here.

Referred by:

____

Include relevant vital sign measurements as medical personnel complete your evaluation. (Reference key on page xi.)

BP __________   HR__________   Tp __________   Rp __________

HT __________   Wt__________   GL __________   Ch __________

Other ____

____

Diagnosis

____

____

____

____

____

____

____

Actions Needed *(follow-up, referral, prescriptions, tests, etc.)*   Date Scheduled

____

____

____

____

Outcome

____

____

____

____

Healthcare Concern/Questions/Symptoms

Date _______________

____

____

____

____

____

____

____

Staple physician's or other healthcare provider's business card or write in contact information here.

Referred by:

____

Include relevant vital sign measurements as medical personnel complete your evaluation. (Reference key on page xi.)

BP __________ HR__________ Tp__________ Rp__________

HT__________ Wt__________ GL__________ Ch__________

Other ____

____

Diagnosis

____

____

____

____

____

____

____

Actions Needed *(follow-up, referral, prescriptions, tests, etc.)*   Date Scheduled

____

____

____

____

Outcome

____

____

____

____

Healthcare Concern/Questions/Symptoms   Date _______________

____

____

____

____

____

____

____

Staple physician's or other healthcare provider's business card or write in contact information here.

Referred by:

____

Include relevant vital sign measurements as medical personnel complete your evaluation. (Reference key on page xi.)

BP __________   HR__________   Tp __________   Rp __________

HT __________   Wt__________   GL __________   Ch __________

Other ___________________________________

____

Diagnosis

____

____

____

____

____

____

____

Actions Needed *(follow-up, referral, prescriptions, tests, etc.)*   Date Scheduled

____

____

____

____

Outcome

____

____

____

____

Healthcare Concern/Questions/Symptoms

Date __________________

____

____

____

____

____

____

Staple physician's or other healthcare provider's business card or write in contact information here.

Referred by:

____

Include relevant vital sign measurements as medical personnel complete your evaluation. (Reference key on page xi.)

BP __________   HR__________   Tp__________   Rp__________

HT__________   Wt__________   GL__________   Ch__________

Other ____

____

Diagnosis

____

____

____

____

____

____

Actions Needed *(follow-up, referral, prescriptions, tests, etc.)*   Date Scheduled

____

____

____

____

Outcome

____

____

____

____

Healthcare Concern/Questions/Symptoms

Date _______________

____

____

____

____

____

____

____

Staple physician's or other healthcare provider's business card or write in contact information here.

Referred by:

____

Include relevant vital sign measurements as medical personnel complete your evaluation. (Reference key on page xi.)

BP _________   HR_________   Tp_________   Rp_________

HT _________   Wt_________   GL _________   Ch_________

Other _______________________________________

____

Diagnosis

____

____

____

____

____

____

Actions Needed *(follow-up, referral, prescriptions, tests, etc.)*

Date Scheduled

____

____

____

____

Outcome

____

____

____

____

Healthcare Concern/Questions/Symptoms

Date _______________

____

____

____

____

____

____

____

____

> *Staple physician's or other healthcare provider's business card or write in contact information here.*
>
> Referred by:
>
> _______________________________________

Include relevant vital sign measurements as medical personnel complete your evaluation. (Reference key on page xi.)

BP __________   HR__________   Tp__________   Rp__________

HT__________   Wt__________   GL__________   Ch__________

Other ____

____

Diagnosis

____

____

____

____

____

____

____

Actions Needed *(follow-up, referral, prescriptions, tests, etc.)*   Date Scheduled

____

____

____

____

Outcome

____

____

____

____

Healthcare Concern/Questions/Symptoms

Date __________________

____

____

____

____

____

____

Include relevant vital sign measurements as medical personnel complete your evaluation. (Reference key on page xi.)

BP __________   HR__________   Tp__________   Rp__________

HT__________   Wt__________   GL__________   Ch__________

Other   _______________________________________

____

Staple physician's or other healthcare provider's business card or write in contact information here.

Referred by:

____

Diagnosis

____

____

____

____

____

____

Actions Needed *(follow-up, referral, prescriptions, tests, etc.)*   Date Scheduled

____

____

____

____

Outcome

____

____

____

____

Healthcare Concern/Questions/Symptoms

Date _________________

____

____

____

____

____

____

Include relevant vital sign measurements as medical personnel complete your evaluation. (Reference key on page xi.)

BP _________   HR_________   Tp_________   Rp_________

HT_________   Wt_________   GL _________   Ch _________

Other _______________________________________

____

Staple physician's or other healthcare provider's business card or write in contact information here.

Referred by:

____

Diagnosis

____

____

____

____

____

____

Actions Needed *(follow-up, referral, prescriptions, tests, etc.)*   Date Scheduled

____

____

____

____

Outcome

____

____

____

____

Personal Healthcare Record for: ____ *Page* __________

Healthcare Concern/Questions/Symptoms

Date _______________

____

____

____

____

____

____

____

Staple physician's or other healthcare provider's business card or write in contact information here.

Referred by:

____

Include relevant vital sign measurements as medical personnel complete your evaluation. (Reference key on page xi.)

BP __________   HR__________   Tp__________   Rp__________

HT __________   Wt__________   GL__________   Ch__________

Other ____

____

Diagnosis

____

____

____

____

____

____

____

Actions Needed *(follow-up, referral, prescriptions, tests, etc.)*   Date Scheduled

____

____

____

____

Outcome

____

____

____

____

Healthcare Concern/Questions/Symptoms

Date ________________

____

____

____

____

____

____

____

Staple physician's or other healthcare provider's business card or write in contact information here.

Referred by:

____

Include relevant vital sign measurements as medical personnel complete your evaluation. (Reference key on page xi.)

BP __________ HR__________ Tp__________ Rp__________

HT__________ Wt__________ GL__________ Ch__________

Other ________________________________

Diagnosis

____

____

____

____

____

____

Actions Needed *(follow-up, referral, prescriptions, tests, etc.)*   Date Scheduled

____

____

____

____

Outcome

____

____

____

____

Healthcare Concern/Questions/Symptoms

Date _______________

____

____

____

____

____

____

____

Include relevant vital sign measurements as medical personnel complete your evaluation. (Reference key on page xi.)

BP __________   HR __________   Tp __________   Rp __________

HT __________   Wt __________   GL __________   Ch __________

Other ____

____

> *Staple physician's or other healthcare provider's business card or write in contact information here.*
>
> Referred by:
>
> ____

Diagnosis

____

____

____

____

____

____

Actions Needed *(follow-up, referral, prescriptions, tests, etc.)*   Date Scheduled

____

____

____

____

Outcome

____

____

____

____

SECTION B

Health History

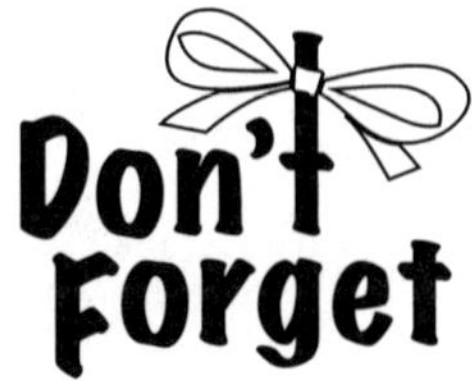

Personal Healthcare Record

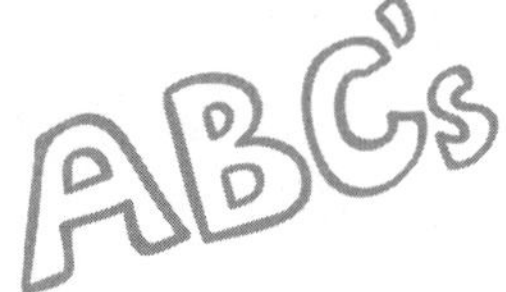

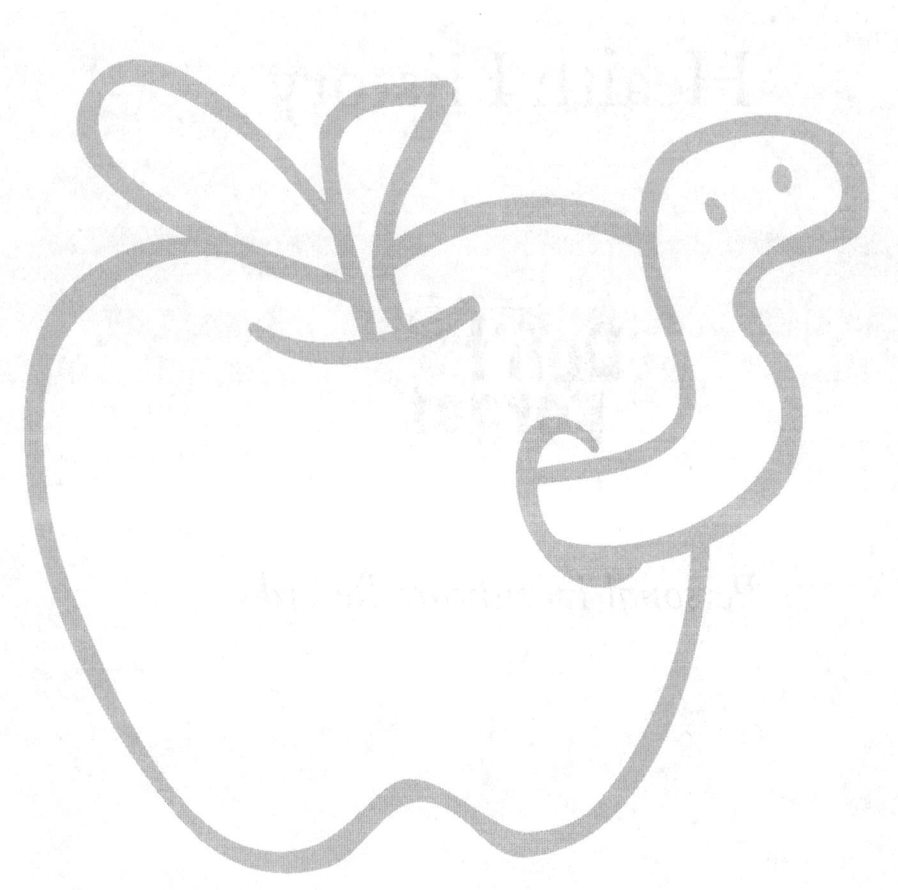

Health History

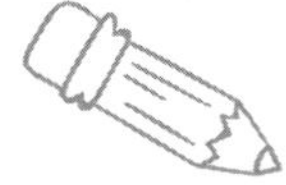

At-a-Glance

 *Note: We strongly recommend putting this page in a protector and placing it at the very beginning of the PHR so it may serve as a quick reference for emergency personnel. See pages 73-94 for detailed Health History information.*

Child's Name _________________________ Home Phone _________________________

Address ____

City, State, Zip ____

Current Photo

Current Medications *include over the counter medications and supplements.* **(see page 76)**

____

____

Current Critical or Chronic Conditions

Note: If you have any of the conditions on page 77, especially conditions noted in BOLD, note them in this section.

Known Allergies (see page 73) ____

____

Drugs ____

____

Food ____

____

Other ____

Emergency Contact(s)

____

Name/Relationship (Parent/Guardian)	Phone – Home	Cell

	Circle		
Authorization for Minor's Medical Treatment	No	Yes	*(see page 70)*
Health Insurance	No	Yes	*(see page 75)*
Religious Preference			
Organ donor	No	Yes	
Contact lenses	No	Yes	
Hearing Aids	No	Yes	
Dentures	No	Yes	
Metal Prosthesis or Implants	No	Yes	Location: _____________

Primary Care Physician _______________ Phone _______________

Note: Continue on back of this page if more space is needed.
Emergency personnel, please photocopy and return this sheet to patient.

Authorization for Minor's Medical Treatment

Insert a signed copy of your child's Authorization for Minor's Medical Treatment (page 109) here.

 Hint: Sign but do not date form until needed for use.

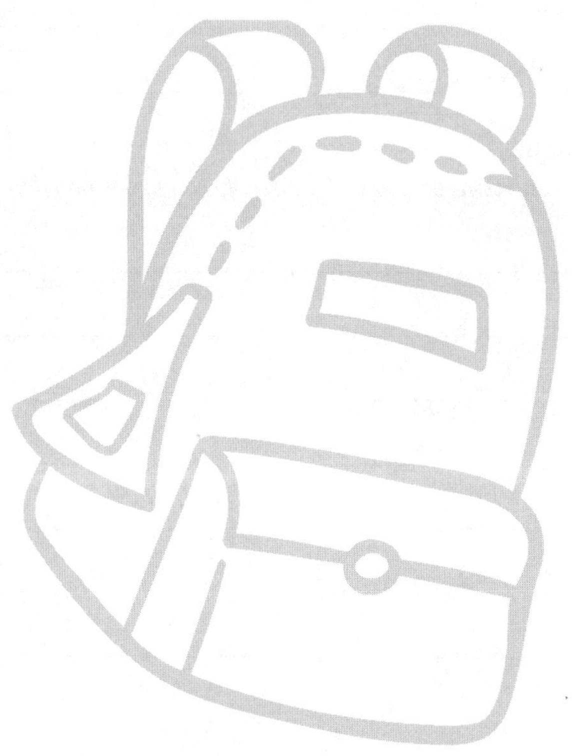

Wallet Card

Complete the wallet card information below and cut out to carry in your wallet for a quick reference. If additional space is needed, make a second card from the template and fold together with the one provided. Review and update information annually or anytime your information changes. Card stock is recommended, but not necessary, for durability.

FRONT

CUT OUT   FOLD HERE   FOLD HERE

MEDICAL INFORMATION

Pharmacy: _______________

Phone: _______________

Surgeries: _______________

____

____

____

Allergies: _______________

____

____

Eye Glass/Contact Perscription:

____

Blood Type: _______________

PHYSICIAN INFORMATION

Physician: _______________

Phone: _______________

Physician: _______________

Phone: _______________

EMERGENCY CONTACT:

Name: _______________

Address: _______________

____

____

Phone: _______________

POCKET REFERENCE

Personal Healthcare Record

Don't Forget

Name _______________

CONFIDENTIAL

If found, please return to Emergency Contact

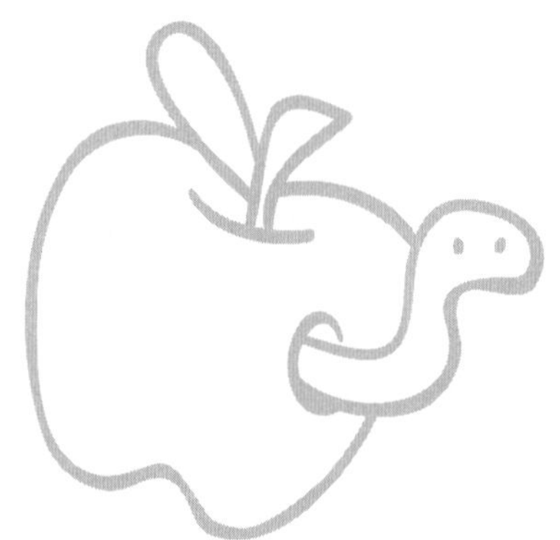

Wallet Card

BACK

MEDICATIONS	DOSAGE	TIMES/ DAY	DATE STARTED	CONDITION

Health History

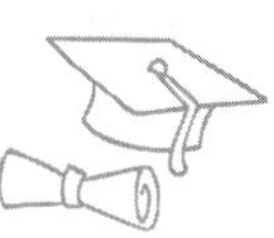

Personal Information

Note: For convenience, the following information can be photocopied and provided to your healthcare provider. Complete any of the information that could change in pencil. Use ink for permanent information. Include this information on your wallet card, too!

Child's Name ________________________________   Home Phone ________________________________

Address ____

City, State, Zip ____

Email Address ____

Blood Type ____

Note: Current Health Care Provider information is listed on each journal page and on page 74.

Known Allergies

Name of Drug, Food, Plant, Other	Typical Reactions Comments, Treatment	First Developed

Religious Preference: ____

Emergency Contact(s)

Name ________________________________   Home Phone ________________________________

Address ________________________________   Cell ________________________________

City, State, Zip ____

Authorization to Treat (Child)

Note: A copy of your child's Authorization for Minor's Medical Treatment or Authorization to Treat is located on page 70

Date Completed ________________________________   Location ________________________________

Health Insurance

 *Hint: Copy the front and back of all current insurance cards and keep these copies in your PHR. We also recommend getting signed Insurance Verification forms from any new healthcare professionals you may visit (see Template/Section page 111).*

Primary Insurance Company ____

Group/Policy Number ______________________ Member ID Number ___________________________

Address ____ Phone ___________________________

____

Member Name ____

Secondary Insurance Company ____

Group/Policy Number ______________________ Member ID Number ___________________________

Address ____ Phone ___________________________

____

Member Name ____

Prescription Drug Service ____

Group/Policy Number ______________________ Member ID Number ___________________________

Address ____ Phone ___________________________

____

Member Name ____

Other Insurance Information

____

____

____

____

Medications

Medications	Dosage	Times/Day	Date Started	Condition

Common Health Conditions

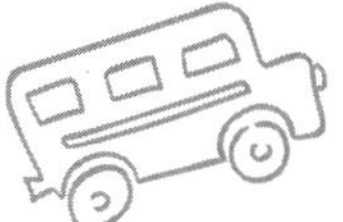

Indicate if your child has or has in the past been diagnosed with any of the following by placing a date or approximate date the problem began.

Health Condition	Date Began	Health Condition	Date Began
Acid reflux		Hypertension	
AIDS, AIDS related disorders		Insomnia	
Angina		Kidney disease	
Anxiety		Liver disease	
Aneurysm		Meningitis	
Arrhythmia		Mental/Nervous Disorders	
Arthritis		Migraine	
Asthma		Muscular dystrophy	
Back Pain		Musculoskeletal/joint problems	
Bipolar disorder		Myocardial infarction	
Bleeding or blood disorder		Nasal polyps	
Blood clots and VTE		Nausea, gas, indigestion	
Bronchitis		Pancreas	
Cancer		Peptic ulcer	
Chest pain		Rectal problems	
Chronic obstructive pulmonary disease (COPD)		Rhinitis	
Constipation, loose bowels, diarrhea		Rheumatic fever	
Cystic fibrosis		Shortness of breath	
Depression		Sinusitis	
Diabetes		Sleeping problems	
Dizziness		Stomach problems	
Endocrine problems		Tired, unusually	
Epilepsy		Tuberculosis	
Fainting spells		Tumor	
Gall bladder		Other – list below	
Gastroesophageal reflux disease (GERD/GORD)			
Hay fever			
Headaches			
Heart attack			
Heart failure			
Heart murmur			
Heartburn			
Hernia			
High blood pressure			
High cholesterol			

Early Childhood

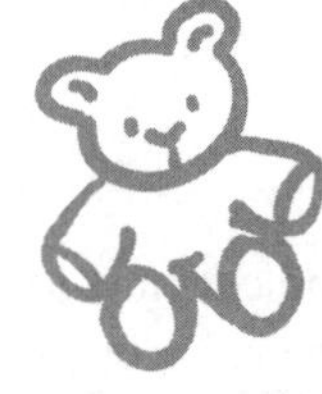

Birth

Date _______________________ Time _______________________

Weight _______________ *(Percentile__________)*   Length_______________ *(Percentile__________)*

Hair Color _______________ Eye Color _______________   Head Circumference__________ *(Percentile__________)*

Location ____   Doctor_________________________________

Address ____

Condition of health at birth: (circle one)   Normal   Complications

APGAR Scores: 1 minute_______________   5 minutes _______________

Complications? Please describe. ____

____

____

____

____

____

____

____

____

____

____

____

____

____

____

____

Important Healthcare Event Reminders & Checklist

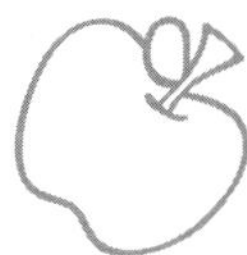

Birth to age 12 Your doctor(s) will guide you through these years, concentrating primarily on bodily functions, developmental activities and immunizations. For more detailed information, see your doctor or any of the resources listed.

Age 13 to 17 Physicals for sports activities begin about this time. General health factors including height, weight, blood pressure will be checked. If concerns are present, see your doctor as you would for any other medical condition. Additionally, for girls, doctors recommend a gynecological exam conducted by an obstetrician-gynecologist (OB/GYN) between ages of 13-15 or when they become sexually active whichever comes first. (Advice on how to handle this first appointment is available from a number of resources including your doctor.) Self-exams of breast should begin. Pap Smear exams should begin if concerns are present.

Development

Date	The Firsts	Comments
	Feeding (breast or bottle)	
	Turning Over	
	Crawling	
	Word (What was it?)	

Vaccinations and Immunizations

Shots/Other Procedures	Site on Body	Reactions/Results	Action

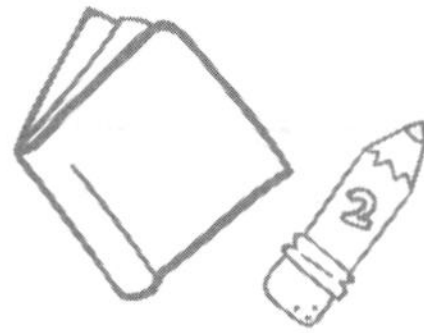

Update for Biological Parent and Sibling Health Summary

Health of Parents, Siblings, Blood Relatives

Hint: Note Date Updated *(Recommend annually or if any major changes occur.)* ______________________

____

Biological Mother: Date of birth ___________________ Name ___________________________________

If living, condition of health :   excellent   good   fair   poor   Male   Female

Why?____

____

____

____

Major health concerns: ____

____

____

____

If deceased, age __________   Cause of death ____

Biological Father: Date of birth ___________________ Name ___________________________________

If living, condition of health :   excellent   good   fair   poor   Male   Female

Why?____

____

____

Major health concerns: ____

____

____

____

If deceased, age __________   Cause of death ____

 *Hint: If needed, before completing this page, make additional pages for additional family members.*

Biological Sibling: Date of birth ________________ Name ________________

If living, condition of health :   excellent   good   fair   poor   Male   Female

Why? ________________

____

Major health concerns: ________________

____

If deceased, age __________ Cause of death ________________

Biological Sibling: Date of birth ________________ Name ________________

If living, condition of health :   excellent   good   fair   poor   Male   Female

Why? ________________

____

Major health concerns: ________________

____

If deceased, age __________ Cause of death ________________

Biological Sibling: Date of birth ________________ Name ________________

If living, condition of health :   excellent   good   fair   poor   Male   Female

Why? ________________

____

Major health concerns: ________________

____

If deceased, age __________ Cause of death ________________

Biological Mother's Side

 *Hint: If needed, before completing this page, make additional pages for additional family members.*

(Other blood relatives who have/had critical medical conditions grandparents, aunts, uncles.)

Relationship _________________________   Name _____________________________________

Date of birth _________________________

If living, condition of health :   excellent   good   fair   poor   Male   Female

Why? ____

____

Major health concerns: ____

____

If deceased, age _____________   Cause of death ___________________________________

Relationship _________________________   Name _____________________________________

Date of birth _________________________

If living, condition of health :   excellent   good   fair   poor   Male   Female

Why? ____

____

Major health concerns: ____

____

If deceased, age _____________   Cause of death ___________________________________

Relationship _________________________   Name _____________________________________

Date of birth _________________________

If living, condition of health :   excellent   good   fair   poor   Male   Female

Why? ____

____

Major health concerns: ____

____

If deceased, age _____________   Cause of death ___________________________________

Biological Father's Side

 *Hint: If needed, before completing this page, make additional pages for additional family members.*

(Other blood relatives who have/had critical medical conditions grandparents, aunts, uncles.)

Relationship _______________________   Name ____

Date of birth _______________________

If living, condition of health :   excellent   good   fair   poor   Male   Female

Why? ____

____

Major health concerns: ____

____

If deceased, age _________   Cause of death _____________________________________

Relationship _______________________   Name ____

Date of birth _______________________

If living, condition of health :   excellent   good   fair   poor   Male   Female

Why? ____

____

Major health concerns: ____

____

If deceased, age _________   Cause of death _____________________________________

Relationship _______________________   Name ____

Date of birth _______________________

If living, condition of health :   excellent   good   fair   poor   Male   Female

Why? ____

____

Major health concerns: ____

____

If deceased, age _________   Cause of death _____________________________________

Surgeries or Hospitalizations
(Serious Illness or Injury)

 *Note: See Page 77 for a list of common diseases*

Date	Illness or Injury

Vaccinations and Immunizations

Hint: Consult your physician for direction. Other references:
Centers for Disease Control and Prevention http://www.cdc.gov
American Academy of Pediatrics at http://www.aap.org

Birth – 17 Years

Vaccine	Defined	Date Given	Type of Vaccine	Site on Body/ Reactions	Doctor's Office or Clinic	Date Next Dose Due
	OPV – oral polio virus IPV – injectable polio virus					
Polio 1						
Polio 2						
Polio 3						
Polio 4						
DTP, Td, DT 1	diphtheria, tetanus, acellular pertussis DTap, Tdap					
DTP, Td, DT 2						
DTP, Td, DT 3						
DTP, Td, DT 4						
DTP, Td, DT 5						
Rota	Rotavirus Gastroenteritis - diarrhea					

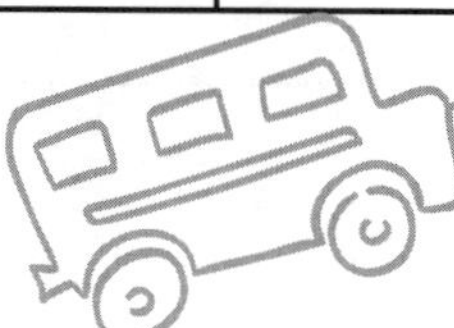

Vaccine	Defined	Date Given	Type of Vaccine	Site on Body/ Reactions	Doctor's Office or Clinic	Date Next Dose Due
MMR 1	mumps, measles, rubella					
MMR 2						
Varicella	chicken pox					
Hib	homophilus influenza type B					
MCV4	meningococcal meningitis					
Hep A	hepatitis type A virus					
Hep B 1	hepatitis type B virus					
Hep B 2						
Hep B 3						
TB Skin Test 1	tuberculosis					
TB Skin Test 1						
PCV	ear infections, meningitis, pneumonia, and septicemia					
HPV	human papilloma virus					
Influenza Vaccine	flu (annual)					
Zoster	Shingles					

Hospitalizations
(Other)

 *Note: Include this information on the wallet card.*

Date	Reason for Hospitalization

Dental Records

(Optional quick cross reference for Journal pages)

Date	Purpose of Visit

Hearing Records

(Optional quick cross reference for Journal pages)

Date	Purpose of Visit	Results

Vision Records

(Optional quick cross reference for Journal pages)

Date	Purpose of Visit	Results Without Correction/With Correction

Development and Identification Photographs

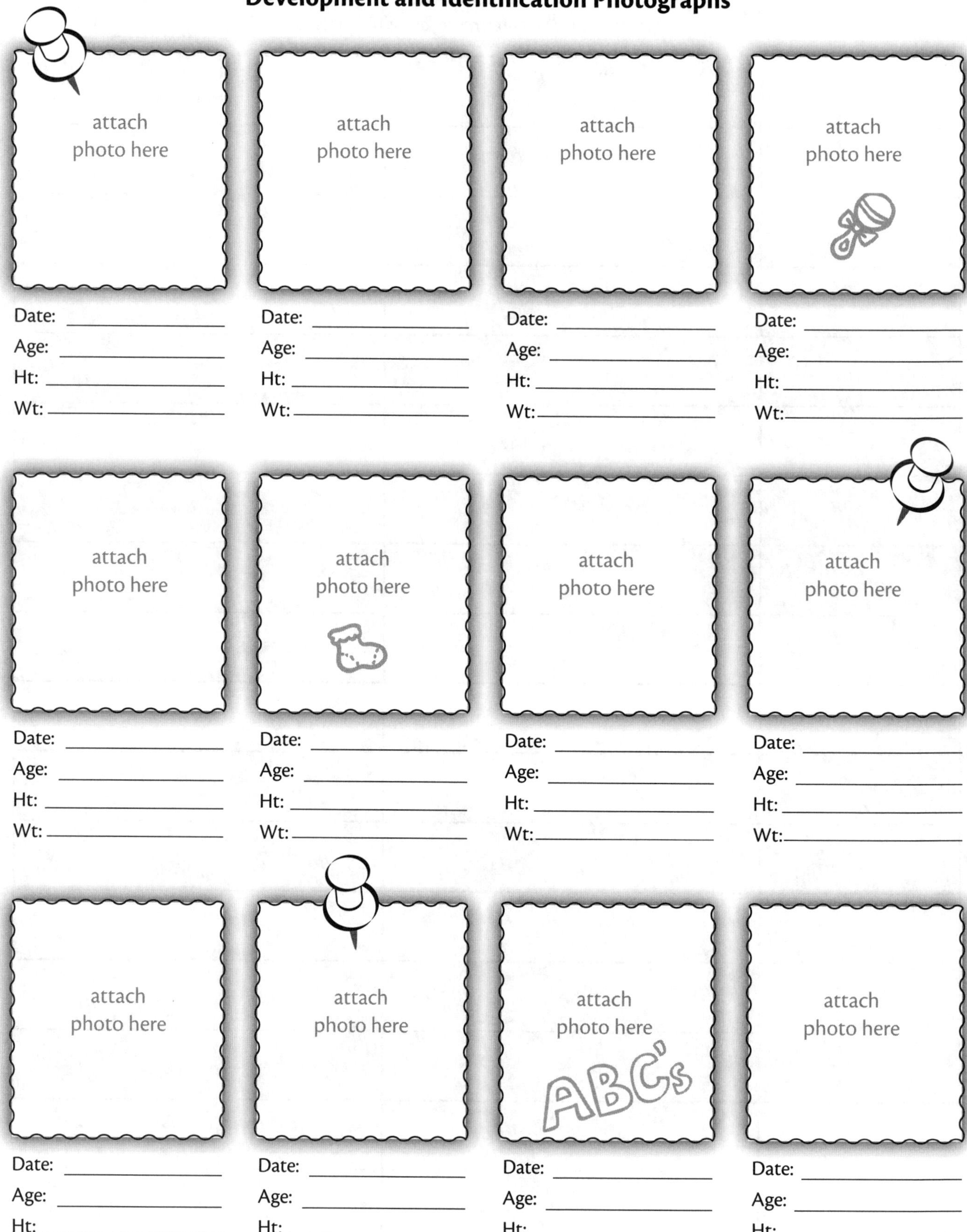

attach photo here

Date: ___________
Age: ___________
Ht: ___________
Wt: ___________

attach photo here

Date: ___________
Age: ___________
Ht: ___________
Wt: ___________

attach photo here

Date: ___________
Age: ___________
Ht: ___________
Wt: ___________

attach photo here

Date: ___________
Age: ___________
Ht: ___________
Wt: ___________

attach photo here

Date: ___________
Age: ___________
Ht: ___________
Wt: ___________

attach photo here

Date: ___________
Age: ___________
Ht: ___________
Wt: ___________

attach photo here

Date: ___________
Age: ___________
Ht: ___________
Wt: ___________

attach photo here

Date: ___________
Age: ___________
Ht: ___________
Wt: ___________

attach photo here

Date: ___________
Age: ___________
Ht: ___________
Wt: ___________

attach photo here

Date: ___________
Age: ___________
Ht: ___________
Wt: ___________

attach photo here

Date: ___________
Age: ___________
Ht: ___________
Wt: ___________

attach photo here

Date: ___________
Age: ___________
Ht: ___________
Wt: ___________

Development and Identification Photographs

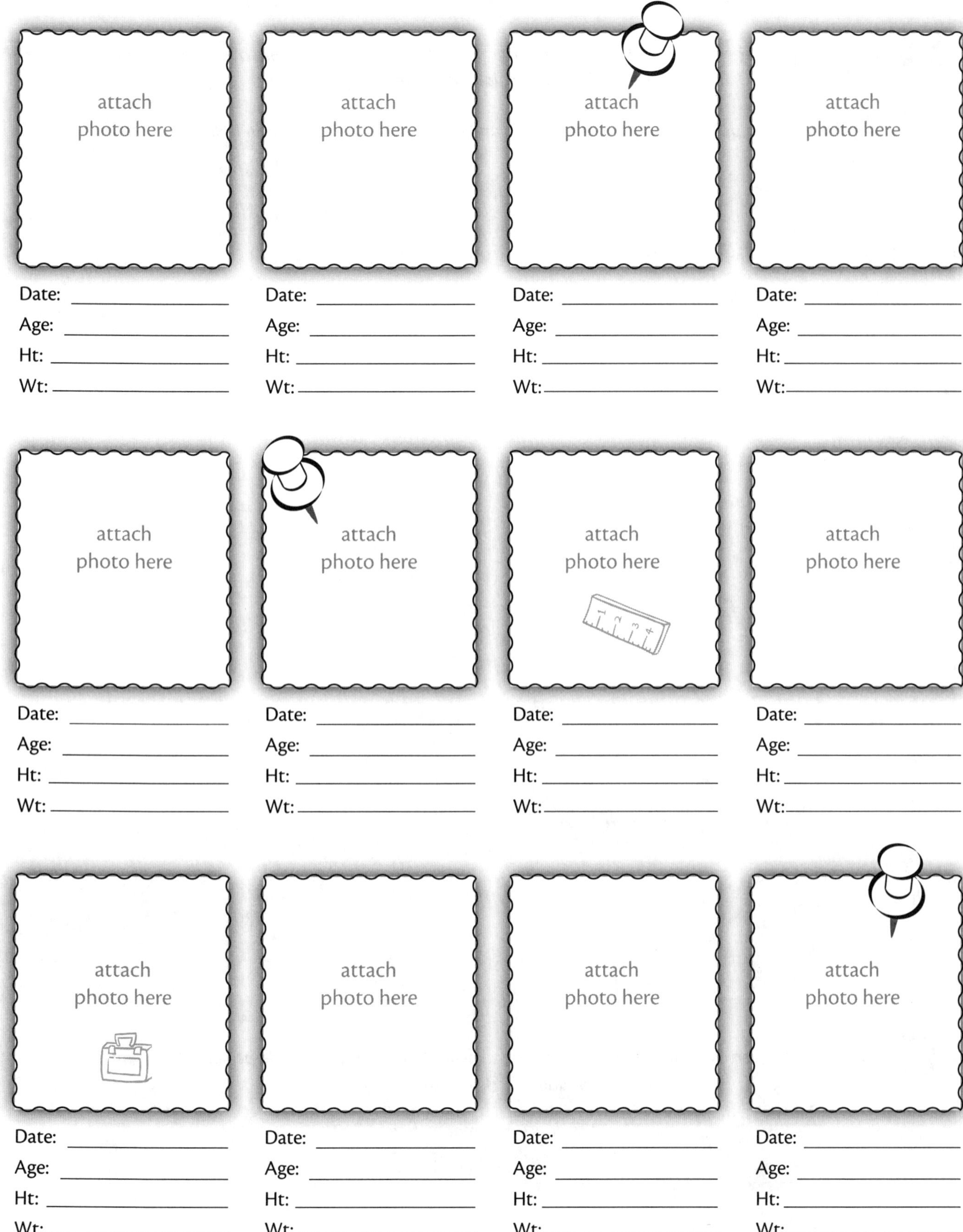

attach photo here	attach photo here	attach photo here	attach photo here
Date: __________	Date: __________	Date: __________	Date: __________
Age: __________	Age: __________	Age: __________	Age: __________
Ht: __________	Ht: __________	Ht: __________	Ht: __________
Wt: __________	Wt: __________	Wt: __________	Wt: __________

Identification Records

 *Note: Attach finger print records to this page. Finger printing can be obtained from a variety of locations. Check with your local law enforcement agency.*

 *Note: Insert hair clippings in a small plastic baggie and attach to this page for use in DNA tests, if needed.*

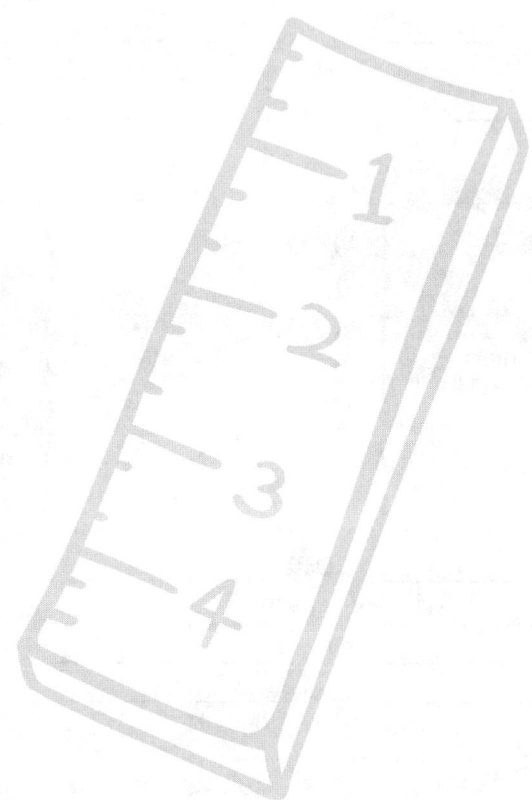

 *Note: Amber Alert Personal Tracking Devices are available for use in your child's personal belongings. For more information check www.amberalertgps.com*

List device information here.

____

____

SECTION C

Healthcare Reference Information

*A section where you can add additional healthcare articles
and information, specific to your child's needs.*

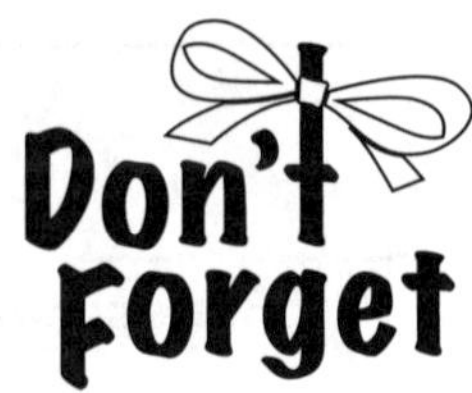

The contents of the Personal Healthcare Record are not designed
to offer medical advice or replace your doctor's healthcare advice or records.

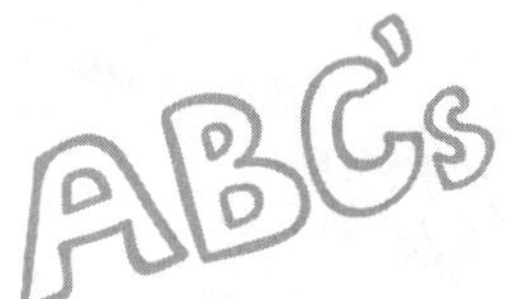

General Range Chart for Common Health Indicators

Individual health conditions vary. The general information provided below, obtained from a variety of public sources, may change due to continued research. The websites listed on page 101 may be consulted for more detailed and up-to-date information.

 *Caution:* *The contents of the Personal Healthcare Record are not designed to offer medical advice or replace your doctor's healthcare advice or records.*

	Normal/Average Range		
Temperature	97.8 – 99.1 degrees Fahrenheit / average 98.6 degrees Fahrenheit		
Breathing	12-18 breaths per minute		
Blood Pressure	**Adults** *mm of mercury (mm Hg)*	**Systolic** *(top number)*	**Diastolic** *(bottom number)*
	Normal	Less than 120	And Less than 80
	Prehypertension	120–139	Or 80–89
	High Blood Pressure		
	Stage 1	140–159	Or 90–99
	Stage 2	160 or higher	Or 100 or higher

		Beats per minute (resting)
Pulse/Heart Rate		
	Newborn Infants	100 - 160
	Children 1 – 10 years	70 -100
	Over 10 Years *(includes adults and seniors)*	60 – 100
	Well-trained Athletes	40 – 60
	Exercise Heart Rate	Exercise 60-90% of your maximum heart rate. To determine you maximum heart rate. Subtract your age from 220 to get your beats per minute. Multiply your beats per minute by 0.6 and again by 0.9 to get your personal range.

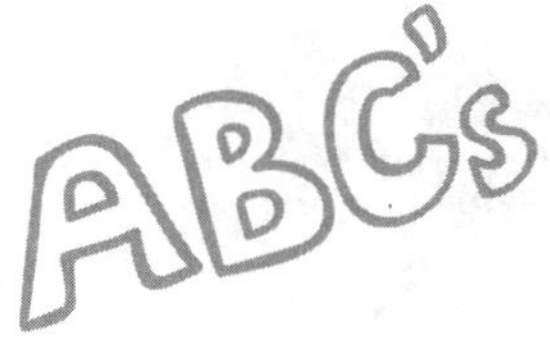

LDL (Bad) Cholesterol	mg/dL	
	Optimal	Less than 100
	Near Optimal/ Above Optimal	100 - 129
	Borderline High	130 - 159
	High	160 - 189
	Very High	190 and above

HDL (Good) Cholesterol	**Average range in mg/dL** *(higher the better)*	
	Men	40 – 50
	Women	50 – 60

Triglyceride Level	mg/dL	
	Normal	Less than 150
	Borderline High	150 - 199
	High	200 - 499
	Very High	500

Blood Glucose	**Target Blood Glucose Levels for people with Diabetes**	
	Before meals	70 - 130
	1 – 2 hours after start of meal	less than 180
	Low Blood Glucose (Hypoglycemia)	below 70

Weight	**Body Mass Index (BMI)**	
	Healthy	18.5 – 24.9
	Overweight	25 – 29.9
	Obese	30 or greater
	Or consult standard height/weight charts	

2 to 20 years: Boys
Stature-for-age and Weight-for-age percentiles

NAME _______________________

RECORD # _______________

Mother's Stature _____________ Father's Stature _____________

Date	Age	Weight	Stature	BMI*

***To Calculate BMI**: Weight (kg) ÷ Stature (cm) ÷ Stature (cm) x 10,000
or Weight (lb) ÷ Stature (in) ÷ Stature (in) x 703

AGE (YEARS)

12 13 14 15 16 17 18 19 20

STATURE

WEIGHT

95 90 75 50 25 10 5

Published May 30, 2000 (modified 11/21/00).
SOURCE: Developed by the National Center for Health Statistics in collaboration with
the National Center for Chronic Disease Prevention and Health Promotion (2000).
http://www.cdc.gov/growthcharts

CDC

SAFER • HEALTHIER • PEOPLE™

2 to 20 years: Girls
Stature-for-age and Weight-for-age percentiles

NAME _______________________

RECORD # _______________________

Mother's Stature		Father's Stature		
Date	Age	Weight	Stature	BMI*

***To Calculate BMI**: Weight (kg) ÷ Stature (cm) ÷ Stature (cm) x 10,000
or Weight (lb) ÷ Stature (in) ÷ Stature (in) x 703

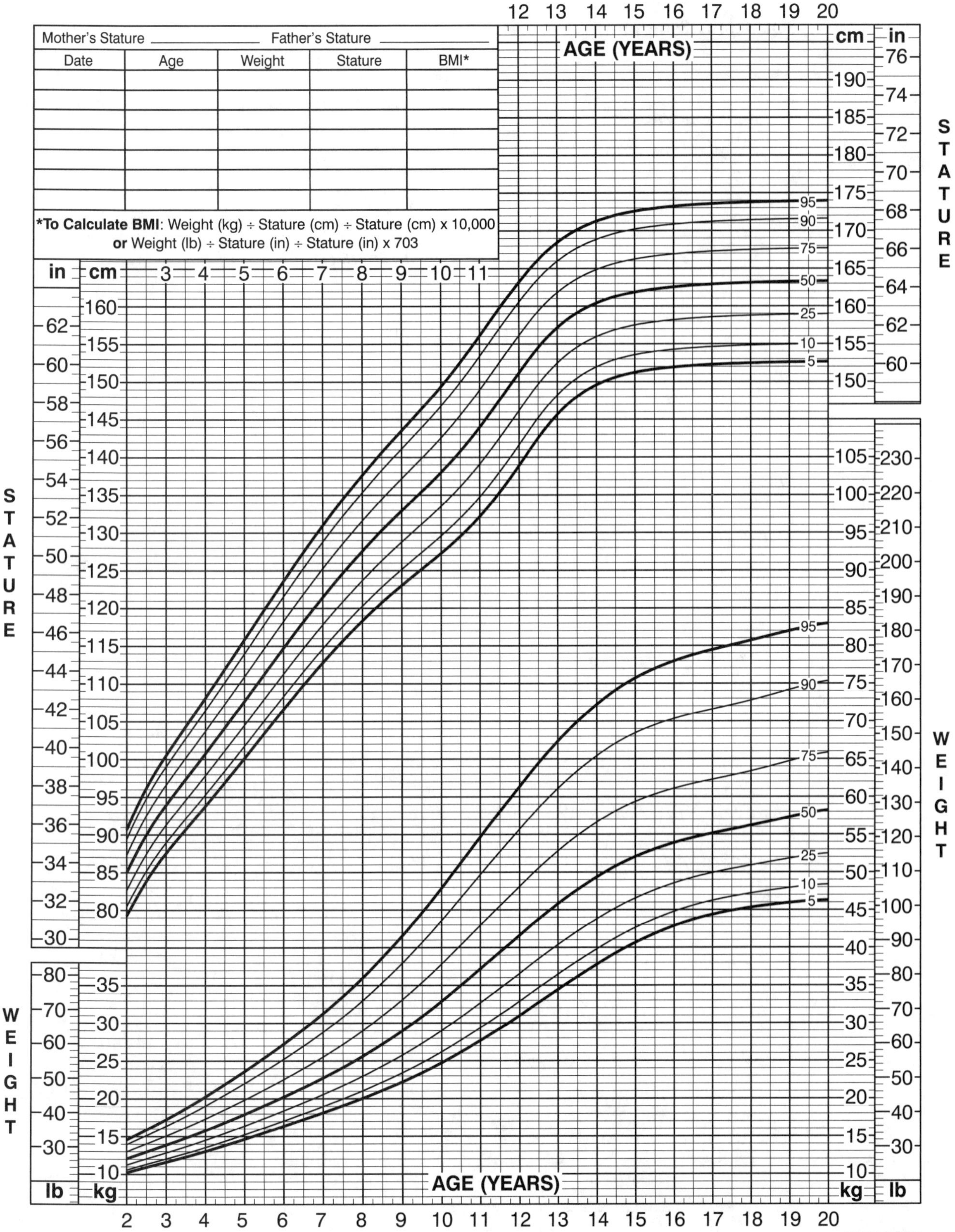

AGE (YEARS)

STATURE

WEIGHT

95
90
75
50
25
10
5

Published May 30, 2000 (modified 11/21/00).
SOURCE: Developed by the National Center for Health Statistics in collaboration with
the National Center for Chronic Disease Prevention and Health Promotion (2000).
http://www.cdc.gov/growthcharts

CDC

SAFER · HEALTHIER · PEOPLE™

Personal Healthcare Record for: _"Journal Page Sample"_   Page __10__

Healthcare Concern/Questions/Symptoms

Date __1/5/XX__

Re-occurring headache

> Staple physician's or other healthcare provider's business card or write in contact information here.
>
> Dr. John Doe
> 123 Any Pl.
> Anytown, State 12345
> 123-456-7890
>
> Referred by: ______________________

Include relevant measurements as medical personnel complete your evaluation.

BP __80/120__ HR________ Tp __99.2__ Rp________

HT __5'8"__ Wt __130__ GL________ Ch________

Other ______________________

Diagnosis

Sinus Infection

Actions Needed *(follow-up, referral, prescriptions, tests, etc.)*   Date Scheduled

1. Perscription for XYZ Antibiotic sent to pharmacy

2. Follow-up appt in 2 weeks   1/22/XX

Outcome

Treatment started- call if any problems

Web-based Medical Information Resources

 *Note: You may need to search through some websites to find the specific information you need, but most websites have built-in search capabilities to help you.*

Amber Alert Child Location GPS System	http://www.amberalertgps.com
American Cancer Society	http://www.cancer.org
American Dental Association	http://www.ada.org/public
American Diabetes Association	http://www.diabetes.org
American Foundation for the Blind	http://www.afb.org
American Heart Association	http://www.americanheart.org
American Medical Association	http://www.ama-assn.org
Department of Health and Human Services & Center for Disease Control & Prevention	http://www.hhs.gov http://www.cdc.gov
National Association for the Deaf	http://www.nad.org
National Institutes of Health & National Library of Medicine On-line Service of NIH	http://www.nih.gov http://www.nlm.nih.gov http://www.medlineplus.gov
National Mental Health Information Center	http://www.mentalhealth.samhsa.gov
National Organization on Disability	http://www.nod.org
Nemours Foundation (Children's Health)	http://www.kidshealth.org
Web MD (General Medical Information)	http://www.webmd.com

Add your own

____

____

____

____

____

____

____

____

Template Pages

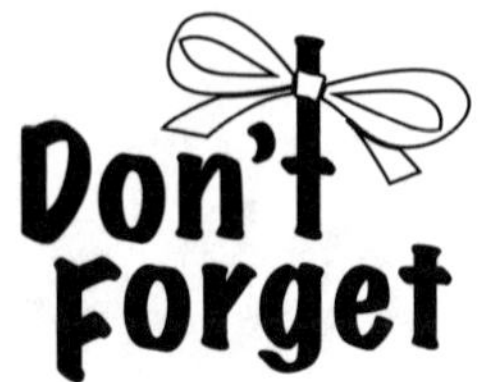

Photocopy Masters
Do Not Write on These Copies

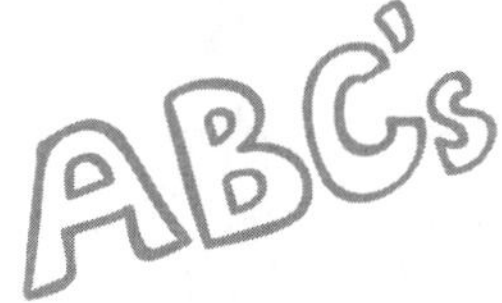

Healthcare Concern/Questions/Symptoms

Date __________________

> Staple physician's or other healthcare provider's business card or write in contact information here.
>
> Referred by:
>
> ___________________________________

Include relevant measurements as medical personnel complete your evaluation.

BP __________   HR __________   Tp __________   Rp __________

HT __________   Wt __________   GL __________   Ch __________

Other ___________________________________

Diagnosis

Actions Needed *(follow-up, referral, prescriptions, tests, etc.)*

Date Scheduled

Outcome

Healthcare Concern/Questions/Symptoms

Date __________________

____

____

____

____

____

____

____

____

> *Staple physician's or other healthcare provider's business card or write in contact information here.*
>
> Referred by:
>
> _______________________________

Include relevant measurements as medical personnel complete your evaluation.

BP __________   HR __________   Tp __________   Rp __________

HT __________   Wt __________   GL __________   Ch __________

Other _______________________________

____

Diagnosis

____

____

____

____

____

____

Actions Needed *(follow-up, referral, prescriptions, tests, etc.)*   Date Scheduled

____

____

____

Outcome

____

____

____

____

Wallet Card

Instructions: *Photo copy card back to back for 2-sided card*

Complete the wallet card information below and cut out to carry in your wallet for a quick reference. If additional space is needed, make a second card from the template and fold together with the one provided. Review and update information annually or anytime your information changes. Card stock is recommended, but not necessary, for durability.

FRONT

CUT OUT   FOLD HERE   FOLD HERE

MEDICAL INFORMATION

Pharmacy: _______________________

Phone: _______________________

Surgeries: _______________________

____

____

____

Allergies: _______________________

____

____

Eye Glass/Contact Perscription:

____

Blood Type: _______________________

PHYSICIAN INFORMATION

Physician: _______________________

Phone: _______________________

Physician: _______________________

Phone: _______________________

EMERGENCY CONTACT:

Name: _______________________

Address: _______________________

____

____

Phone: _______________________

POCKET REFERENCE

Personal Healthcare Record

Don't Forget

Name _______________________

CONFIDENTIAL

If found, please return to Emergency Contact

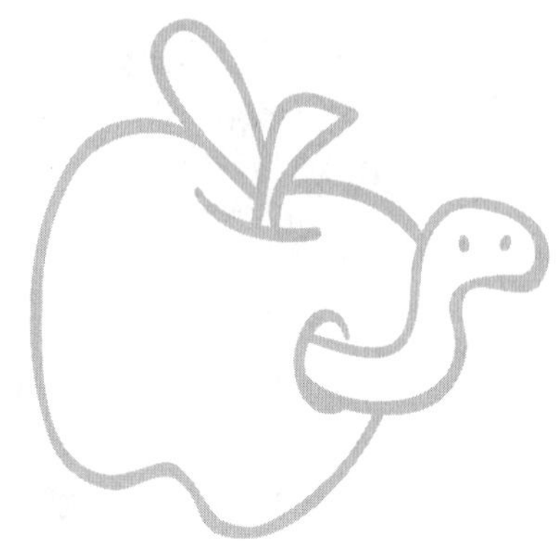

Wallet Card
(Note: Photo copy card back to back for 2-sided card.)

BACK

MEDICATIONS	DOSAGE	TIMES/ DAY	DATE STARTED	CONDITION

AUTHORIZATION FOR MINOR'S MEDICAL TREATMENT

Child's Full Legal Name ____

Date of Birth _________________________ Age ___________ Gender _________________

Doctor's Information

Doctor's Name ____

Doctor's Address ____

Doctor's Office Phone _______________ Doctor's Emergency Phone ___________________

Medical Insurer/Health Plan _______________ Policy # _______________________

Allergies to Medications ____

Allergies (Other) ____

If applicable, please note the conditions for which the child is currently receiving treatment

____

Note any other significant medical information

____

____

____

Dentist's Info

Dentist's Name ____

Dentist's Address ____

Dentist's Office Phone _______________ Dentist's Emergency Phone __________________

Dentist's Insurer/Health Plan _______________ Policy # ____________________

Parent(s)/Legal Guardian(s)

Parent #1 Name ____

Address____

Homephone___________________________ Workphone______________________

Cellphone____________________________ Pager_________________________

Email____

Additional Contact Information__________________________________

____

Parent #2 Name ____

Address____

Homephone___________________________ Workphone______________________

Cellphone____________________________ Pager_________________________

Email____

Additional Contact Information__________________________________

____

Alternate contact in the event Parent(s)/Legal Guardian(s) cannot be reached:

Name____

Address____

Homephone___________________________ Workphone______________________

Cellphone____________________________ Pager_________________________

Email____

Additional Contact Information__________________________________

____

AUTHORIZATION AND CONSENT OF PARENT(S) OR LEGAL GUARDIAN(S)

I do hereby solemnly swear that I have legal custody of the aforementioned minor child.

I grant my authorization and consent for _______________________________________ (hereafter "Supervising Adult") to administer general first aid treatment for any minor injuries or illnesses experienced by the minor. If the injury or illness is life threatening or in need of emergency treatment, I authorize the Supervising Adult to summon any and all professional emergency personnel to attend, transport, and treat the participant and to issue consent for any X-ray, anesthetic, blood transfusion, medication, or other medical diagnosis, treatment, or hospital care deemed advisable by, and to be rendered under the general supervision of, any licensed physician, surgeon, dentist, hospital, or other medical professional or institution duly licensed to practice in the state in which such treatment is to occur.

It is understood that this authorization is given in advance of any such medical treatment, but is given to provide authority and power on the part of the Supervising Adult in the exercise of his or her best judgment upon the advice of any such medical or emergency personnel.

This authorization is effective commencing on the _______ day of _______________________, 20______ and expiring on

the _______________ day of _____________________, 20_____.

Signed this _______ day of___________________, 20 _____.

____

Parent #1 Signature

____

Parent #2 Signature

Certificate of Acknowledgement of Notary Public

STATE OF ___________________

COUNTY OF _________________

This document was acknowledged before me on _______________________ [date]

by ____ [name of principal].

[Notary Seal, if any]

____

(Signature of Notarial Officer)

Notary Public for the State of ________________

My commission expires ____________________

INSURANCE VERIFICATION FORM

Name of Healthcare Professional ____

Business/Clinic Name ____

Address ____

City/State/Zip ____

Phone _______________________   Email _______________________________________

The above healthcare professional is responsible for verifying the insurance coverage accepted by his/her office and notifying the patient, in advance of providing services, if the charges will not be covered or are greater than the reasonable and customary charges accepted by the patient's insurance company. The patient will not be held responsible for any charges not communicated prior to services.

____

Date   Signature of Healthcare Professional

SYMPTOM/HEALTHCARE EVENT JOURNAL

(Optional supplement to journal page for detail of major healthcare events or diary of symptoms and responses to treatments.)

____

____

____

____

____

____

____

____

____

____

____

____

____

____

____

____

____

____

____

____

____

Personal Healthcare Record

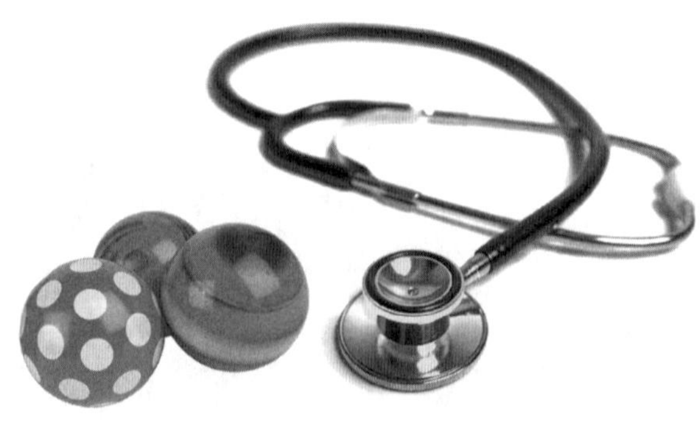

BIRTH TO SEVENTEEN YEARS OLD

For _______________________________
Name

From ___________ *to* ___________
Date   Date

CONFIDENTIAL

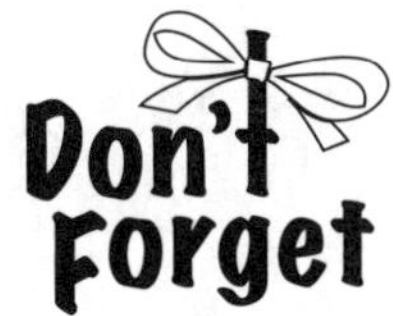

Note: The templates, on the previous page and this page, are to be copied for additional 3 ring view-type notebook inserts, if needed.

Personal Healthcare Record for: _______________

From ______ to ______

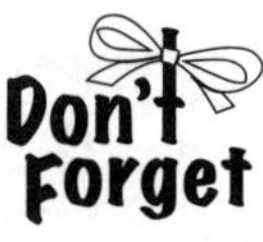

Take charge of your healthcare with the
Personal Healthcare Record

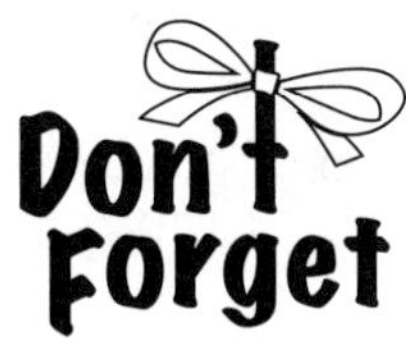

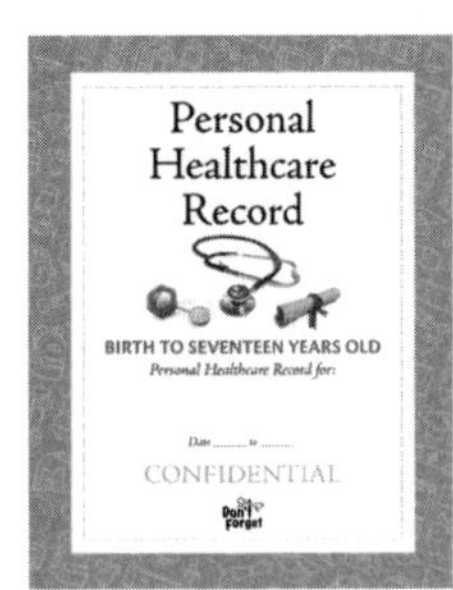

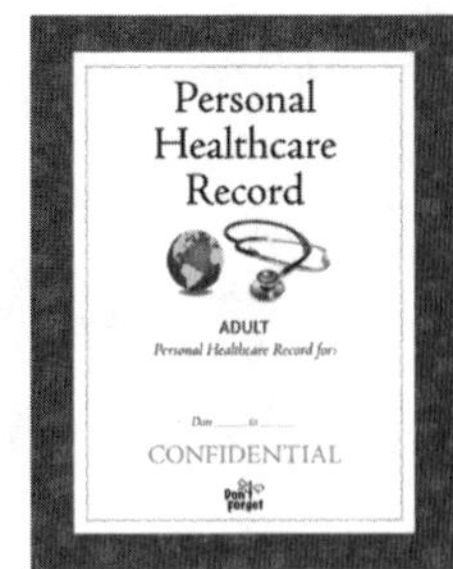

Age Appropriate Content	Birth - 17	Adult (18+)
Healthcare Journal Pages	✓	✓
Health History Including: medical, dental, hearing, vision	✓	✓
Healthcare Event Reminders	✓	✓
Family Health History Information	✓	✓
Immunization Schedules	✓	✓
Personal Identification Info	✓	✓
Resource Websites	✓	✓
Wallet Card	✓	✓
Templates for additional forms	✓	✓
Authorization to Treat (Child)	✓	
Early Childhood Development	✓	
Growth Charts	✓	
Advance Directive Information		✓
Retail Price (Prices Subject to change without notice)	$19.95	$19.95

Get a lifetime of valuable records (*get both versions!*),
when ordered as a set for **only $34.95!**
Available at www.PersonalHealthcareRecord.com